KT-404-359

250 QUESTIONS FOR THE
MRCPCH
Part 2

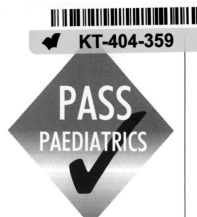

PASS
PAEDIATRICS

WITHDRAWN
FROM LIBRARY

BMA LIBRARY

BRITISH MEDICAL ASSOCIATION

BRITISH MEDICAL ASSOCIATION

0770561

Commissioning Editor: Ellen Green
Development Editor: Helen Leng
Project Manager: Nancy Arnott
Designer: Erik Bigland
Illustration Manager: Bruce Hogarth

250 QUESTIONS FOR THE

MRCPCH
Part 2

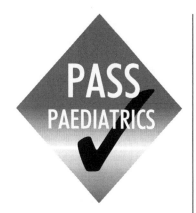

J L Robertson MB ChB MRCPCH

Associate Specialist
Wirral Hospital NHS Trust
Wirral, Merseyside, UK

A P Hughes MB ChB FRCPCH

Consultant Paediatrician
Wirral Hospital NHS Trust
Wirral, Merseyside, UK

SECOND EDITION

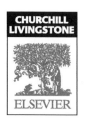

CHURCHILL
LIVINGSTONE

ELSEVIER

EDINBURGH LONDON NEW YORK OXFORD PHILADELPHIA ST LOUIS SYDNEY TORONTO 2006

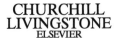

CHURCHILL
LIVINGSTONE
ELSEVIER

© Elsevier Limited 2001
© 2006, Elsevier Limited. All rights reserved.

The right of J L Robertson and A P Hughes to be identified as authors of this work has been asserted by them in accordance with the Copyright, Designs and Patents Act 1988.

No part of this publication may be reproduced, stored in a retrieval system, or transmitted in any form or by any means, electronic, mechanical, photocopying, recording or otherwise, without either the prior permission of the publishers or a licence permitting restricted copying in the United Kingdom issued by the Copyright Licensing Agency, 90 Tottenham Court Road, London W1T 4LP. Permissions may be sought directly from Elsevier's Health Sciences Rights Department in Philadelphia, USA: phone: (+1) 215 239 3804, fax: (+1) 215 239 3805, e-mail: healthpermissions@elsevier.com. You may also complete your request on-line via the Elsevier homepage (http://www.elsevier.com), by selecting 'Customer Support' and then 'Obtaining Permissions'.

First edition 2001

Second edition 2006

ISBN 044310199X

British Library Cataloguing in Publication Data
A catalogue record for this book is available from the British Library

Library of Congress Cataloging in Publication Data
A catalog record for this book is available from the Library of Congress

Note
Knowledge and best practice in this field are constantly changing. As new research and experience broaden our knowledge, changes in practice, treatment and drug therapy may become necessary or appropriate. Readers are advised to check the most current information provided (i) on procedures featured or (ii) by the manufacturer of each product to be administered, to verify the recommended dose or formula, the method and duration of administration, and contraindications. It is the responsibility of the practitioner, relying on his/her own experience and knowledge of the patient, to make diagnoses, to determine dosages and the best treatment for each individual patient, and to take all appropriate safety precautions. To the fullest extent of the law, neither the publisher nor the authors assume any liability for any injury and/or damage to persons or property arising out of or related to any use of the material contained in this book.
The Publisher

Printed in China

ELSEVIER your source for books,
journals and multimedia
in the health sciences

www.elsevierhealth.com

Working together to grow
libraries in developing countries

www.elsevier.com | www.bookaid.org | www.sabre.org

ELSEVIER BOOK AID International Sabre Foundation

Preface

The first edition of this book came about as a result of a single request from one of our SHOs. In preparing for the written section of the MRCPCH Part 2 examination, she asked if we had any data questions that she could use for practice. 'One or two' might have been the initial reply. Instead, however, we started writing down our collection, many of which are real-life scenarios, actually seen and managed in our hospital. These questions started life in a simple format of blocks of 10. Inevitably, however, with our usual desire to explore the limits of opportunity, this very rapidly evolved into a major project, culminating in the first edition.

The second edition has been developed as a result of the college changing the style of the exam. We have written as many of the questions as possible in the new style and added many more.

Some questions we have not been able to rewrite but we believe they are still educational.

J L R
A P H

Contents

Introduction

Answering any exam question is a mixture of knowledge and technique. In our experience, the best technique for answering data questions is as follows:

1. First highlight those parts of the question which you believe are relevant.

2. Then read all the stems of the question, before attempting to answer it.

3. Having answered the question, see if the answers are appropriate for all the highlighted parts.

4. If not, think again – it may be that the answer is wrong; or

5. It may be that certain things underlined are not relevant.

For instance, beware the haematological question with 'Greek child' in it. Thalassaemia may be the correct association, but some Greek children will be iron deficient. The information *may* or *may not* be relevant.

The following example demonstrates the usefulness of this answering system (the italicized words are those you will have highlighted):

1. A 10-day-old female infant presents to you with *vomiting* and *drowsiness*. On examination she is *dehydrated* and has *normal genitalia*:

Sodium	118 mmol/L
Urea	20.8 mmol/L
Glucose	1.8 mmol/L

(a) What is the cause of this child's presenting illness?
  (i) salt-losing crisis
  (ii) inappropriate feeding
  (iii) poor blood sample
  (iv) salt poisoning
  (v) bowel obstruction

(b) What is the underlying diagnosis?
  (i) pyloric stenosis
  (ii) congenital adrenal hyperplasia
  (iii) Munchausen's syndrome by proxy
  (iv) congenital adrenal hypoplasia
  (v) gastroenteritis

You may answer that the child has a salt-losing crisis and congenital adrenal hyperplasia. This may well be right. However, the question specifically says that the baby has *normal* genitalia and therefore the better answer is that of congenital adrenal hypoplasia.

With some questions this will let you know the answer but, if it doesn't, look again. This time, cross out the wrong answers; you will then find you are focusing on only two answers instead of five.

This book is designed to explain *how* to answer the questions, as opposed to explaining the answers. Most of the chapters are divided into five sections:

- Questions (1).
- Answers to questions (1) with brief explanations where relevant.
- Helpful hints. This may need reading several times but will help get you to the answers.

You should now be in a position to answer the second set of questions more appropriately and improve your performance in doing so.

- Questions (2).
- Answers to questions (2).

The book then has three exams. Each should be completed in one sitting before looking at the answer. We have finished with themed and long questions and we have tried to offer advice as to the best way to answer these.

Respiratory medicine

QUESTIONS (1)

1.1 You are asked to review the lung function tests on a nine-year-old boy:

	Predicted	**Measured**	
FVC	2.06	1.30	(63%)
FEV₁	1.86	1.05	(51%)
PEF	272	212	

(a) What type of picture do these results demonstrate?
    (i) restrictive
    (ii) obstructive
    (iii) normal
    (iv) mixed restrictive and obstructive
    (v) poor technique

(b) Give the most likely underlying diagnosis:
    (i) pneumonia
    (ii) asthma
    (iii) muscular dystrophy
    (iv) normal
    (v) croup

1.2 A six-year-old boy is reviewed in your respiratory clinic. He is known to have cystic fibrosis:

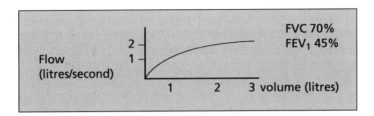

(a) What type of picture do these results demonstrate?
- (i) restrictive
- (ii) obstructive
- (iii) normal
- (iv) mixed restrictive and obstructive
- (v) poor technique

(b) What is an appropriate follow-up test?
- (i) repeat investigation
- (ii) repeat after bronchodilator
- (iii) repeat after one month of DNase
- (iv) no need to do anything
- (v) admit for antibiotics

1.3 A 16-year-old girl has had well-controlled asthma for the past two years. When reviewed in clinic this time, the following test results were found:

	Predicted	Measured
FVC (litres)	3.97	3.02
FEV$_1$ (litres)	3.82	1.72
FEF (25–75%)	4.05	1.08

Suggest two possible explanations.

1.4 The following lung function tests were obtained from a 10-year-old boy with cystic fibrosis before and after a one-month course of treatment:

	Predicted	Measured	1 month later
FVC	2.1	1.21 (57%)	1.59 (76%)
FEV$_1$	1.90	1.00 (53%)	1.25 (65%)
PEF	277	205	197

(a) What is the likely treatment?

(b) What is the percentage rise in FEV$_1$?
  (i)   10
  (ii) 15
  (iii) 20
  (iv) 25
  (v)   50

1.5 These are the lung function tests of a 15-year-old asthmatic girl with exercise intolerance:

	Predicted	Measured
FVC	3.91	3.68
FEV$_1$	3.75	2.96
PEF	471	425

She is on moderate doses of inhaled steroids. Give two possible treatment options.

1.6 Below is a diagram of lung volumes:

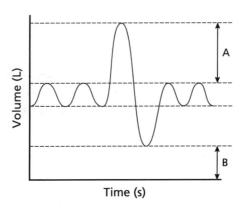

(a) What do the letters A and B represent?
  (i) vital capacity
  (ii) residual volume
  (iii) functional residual capacity
  (iv) expiratory reserve volume
  (v) inspiratory reserve volume
  (vi) tidal volume
  (vii) total lung capacity

(b) Mark the vital capacity (as C) and expiratory reserve volume
  (as D) on the diagram.

1.1 **(a)** (i)

    (b) (iii)
Comment: Both FVC and FEV_1 are markedly reduced. This may also occur in fibrosing alveolitis or fibrosis from other conditions, and in kyphoscoliosis. Note that cystic fibrosis is usually mixed.

1.2 **(a)** (iv)

    (b) (ii)
Comment: FVC is reduced but FEV_1 is reduced by a lot more.

1.3 Poor compliance, smoking or a worsening of her asthma.
The GP had in fact reduced the dose as the patient was well controlled.
Comment: Always put the most likely answer first.

1.4 **(a)** DNase.

    (b) (iv)
Comment: $\dfrac{(1.25 \times 1.00)}{1.00} \times 100 = 25\%.$

1.5 Add an inhaled long-acting beta-agonist, increase the inhaled steroids, or give oral anti-leukotrienes.
Comment: Asthma guidelines.
You do not need to name specific drugs.

1.6 **(a)** A = (v); B = (ii)

(b) Mark the vital capacity (as C) and expiratory reserve volume (as D) on the diagram:

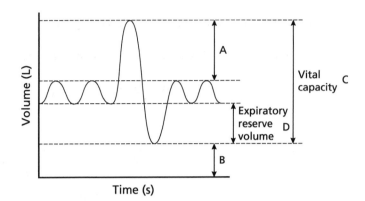

Comment: Remember that one division is always a volume and more than one is always a capacity.

Helpful hints

LUNG FUNCTION TESTS

1. FVC + FEV_1: if both are low this suggests a restrictive picture.

2. FVC near normal with low FEV_1 suggests an obstructive picture.

3. FVC low, but FEV_1 a lot lower suggests a mixed picture.
    For example:

	Predicted	Result (1)	Result (2)	Result (3)
FVC	2.00	1.30↓	1.8→	1.5↓
FEV_1	1.86	1.05↓	1.2↓	1.05 ↓↓
		Restricted	Obstructive	Mixed

4. This may be expressed as a graph with only the percentage predicted for FVC and FEV_1 (e.g. see Question 1.2).

5. The most common restrictive pattern in children is muscular dystrophy and severe scoliosis.

6. The most common obstructive pattern is asthma.

7. CF may be shown as a purely restrictive set of results but is often mixed.

1.7 Draw a diagram of lung volumes showing the following:

A = Vital capacity

B = Functional residual capacity

C = Tidal volume

D = Expiratory reserve volume

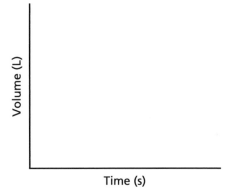

1.8 For the past two winters, a three-year-old child had been noted to suffer from lethargy and coughing which seems to settle each spring. This has been associated with poor feeding. The house is old but not damp and has no central heating. The local authority intervened three weeks ago and the child is now much better.

(a) What is the diagnosis?

(b) What has the council done?

1.9 A 16-year-old boy has been followed up in your clinic for several years. These are his latest lung function tests:

	Predicted	Measured	%
FVC	4.04	3.50	85
FEV$_1$	3.88	2.21	57
PEF	481	253	53
FEF (25–75%)	4.09	1.70	41

(a) What is the diagnosis?
  (i) asthma
  (ii) fibrosing alveolitis
  (iii) muscular dystrophy
  (iv) cystic fibrosis
  (v) bronchiectasis

(b) Which of the above measurements is best for monitoring his condition?
  (i) FVC
  (ii) FEV$_1$
  (iii) PEF
  (iv) FEF (25–75%)
  (v) none of the above

1.10 The following results were found when reviewing a 15-year-old asthmatic girl. She is on inhaled steroids (800 µg b.d.) and a long-acting beta-2 agonist (two puffs b.d.):

	Predicted	Measured	%
FVC	3.97	4.51	114
FEV_1	3.82	3.75	98
PEF	476	491	103
FEF (25–75%)	4.05	3.76	93

What is your management plan?

    (i)   review in 3 months
    (ii) stop the long-acting beta agonist
    (iii) decrease the long acting beta agonist to one puff b.d.
    (iv) decrease the steroids
    (v) stop the steroids

1.11 This seven-year-old has cystic fibrosis and poor exercise tolerance. These are his lung function tests:

FVC	83%	predicted
FEV_1	50%	predicted
FEF (25–75%)	50%	predicted

(a) What test would you do next?

(b) What treatment would you try?

1.12 A nine-year-old boy has asthma. Most of the year he has good control; however, he complains that for the last two weeks the control has been poor. Which of the following tests will best show this?

    (i)   FVC
    (ii) FEV_1
    (iii) peak flow
    (iv) peak flow diary
    (v) FEF (25–75%)

1.13 Causes of hypoxia:

    (i)   hypoventilation
    (ii)   altitude
    (iii) intrapulmonary shunt
    (iv) cardiac shunt
    (v)   adult respiratory distress syndrome
    (vi) pneumonia
    (vii) pure Va/Q mismatch
    (viii) diffusion effect

Which of the above best explain the mechanism of hypoxia below?

(a) You are reviewing a 12-year-old boy in out-patients who you have been following up for the last seven years since being diagnosed as having muscular dystrophy.

(b) You have been caring for a 15-year-old girl who was diagnosed as having Raynaud's at five years. She is then noticed to have increased tightness of the facial skin. You suspect scleroderma.

(c) You are seeing a 10-week-old baby with cyanosis. She seems quite settled and you decide to do an echo. This is normal.

1.14 A seven-year-old is coming up for his three-monthly review. He was diagnosed as having cystic fibrosis four years ago. On questioning, he also has some exercise intolerance which has been helped by the GP prescribing a beta agonist. Which one of the following lung function tests best fits?

	FVC	FEV_1	PEF
Predicted	2.0	1.9	280
(i)	2.2	1.7	210
(ii)	1.6	1.1	200
(iii)	1.5	1.4	170
(iv)	1.7	1.8	250
(v)	1.9	1.0	160

1.15 A 16-year-old has asthma. He is on prophylactic steroids and long-acting beta-2 agonists. You haven't seen him for three months. Which of the following show poor control?

	FVC	FEV$_1$
Predicted	4.00	3.70
(i)	3.90	3.00
(ii)	3.50	3.05
(iii)	2.5	2.3
(iv)	3.00	2.2
(v)	3.60	3.70

1.7

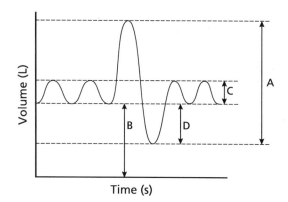

Comment: Remember one space is a volume.

1.8 **(a)** Carbon monoxide poisoning.

(b) Changed the gas heating.
Comment: Nothing else fits all the relevant features – for example, asthma would not usually cause poor feeding.

1.9 **(a)** (i)

(b) (iv)
Comment: FEF (25–75%) is the best measurement for small airway disease. Peak flows are used because of their ease in measurement but they mainly reflect large airways.

1.10 (iv)
Comment: 800 µg b.d. is a high dose and the results showed control.

1.11 **(a)** Bronchodilator response.

(b) Bronchodilators/inhaled steroids/oral steroids.
Comment: FEV_1 and FEF (25–75%) are markedly reduced, suggesting airway obstruction. If there is a bronchodilator response, treatment with bronchodilators plus inhaler or oral steroids may not help.

1.12 (iv)

Comment: Although FEF (25–75%) is the best one-off indicator, the diary is best over time.

1.13 **(a)** (i) **(b)** (viii) **(c)** (iii)

Comment: For learning try to think of a diagnosis to go with all the answers.

1.14 (ii)

Comment: Decide what you would expect the FVC, FEV, PEF should do, then look at the answers.

1.15 (i)

Cardiology

QUESTIONS (1)

2.1 The following are cardiac catheter results in a non-cyanotic 18-month-old child:

	Saturation (%)	Pressure (mmHg)
SVC	79	
RA	88	
RV	86	
PA	86	
LA	96	–/6
LV	96	
A	96	

(a) What is the underlying diagnosis?
- (i) normal
- (ii) ASD
- (iii) Eisenmenger's through an ASD
- (iv) VSD
- (v) Eisenmenger's through a VSD

(b) What pressure would you expect in the right atrium?

2.2 These cardiac catheterization results were obtained on a four-month-old premature baby:

	Saturation (%)
RA	50
RV	50
PA	50
LA	80
LV	80
A	86

(a) Give the most likely diagnosis:
- (i) normal
- (ii) ASD
- (iii) TAPVD
- (iv) chronic lung disease
- (v) acute respiratory illness

(b) What further information do you need to confirm?

2.3 Match the three groups of cardiac lesions to the three syndromes: trisomy 13, 18 and 21.

(a) PDA, septal defects, pulmonary, aortic stenosis.

(b) AVSD, VSD, PDA.

(c) VSD, polyvalvular disease, coronary abnormalities.

2.4 A three-year-old has a cardiac catheterization:

	Saturation (%)	BP
RA	74	–/3
RV	74	70/30
PA	74	25/10
LA	96	
LV	96	

(a) What is the diagnosis?
  (i) PDA
  (ii) pulmonary stenosis
  (iii) ASD
  (iv) pulmonary atresia
  (v) coarctation

(b) Name two changes that may occur on the ECG.

2.5 You are asked to see a six-year-old boy who has seen his GP for headaches. His blood pressure is 150/70. You notice he has a murmur.

(a) What is the most likely diagnosis?
  (i) aortic stenosis
  (ii) PDA
  (iii) renal scarring
  (iv) coarctation
  (v) essential hypertension

(b) Draw a table of approximate pressures and saturations for the left side:

	Saturations	Pressures
LA	96	–/10
LV		
Ascending aorta		
Descending aorta		

ANSWERS (1)

2.1   **(a)** (ii)

(b) −/6.
Comment: Saturations are too high in the right atrium so this is the level of the shunt.

2.2   **(a)** (iv)

(b) Echocardiogram.
Comment: Chronic lung disease is the diagnosis because you would not get Eisenmenger's syndrome through an atrial septal defect by four months.

2.3   **(a)** 18.

(b) 21.

(c) 13.

2.4   **(a)** (ii)

(b) Right ventricular hypertrophy – upright T-wave V_1.
Tall R-wave V_1.
Right axis deviation.
Comment: The saturations are appropriate so it must be a valve problem; therefore look at the pressures.

2.5 **(a)** (iv)

(b)

	Saturations	Pressures
LA	96	–/10
LV	96	150/70
Ascending aorta	96	150/70
Descending abdominal aorta	96	70/30

Comment: An acyanotic lesion, so there is no drop in saturations. The pressures do not have to be precise but there is already one in the question.

Clue to answer **(b)**: include ascending and descending.

Helpful hints

INTERPRETATION OF CARDIAC CATHETERIZATION

Draw a schematic heart. For example:

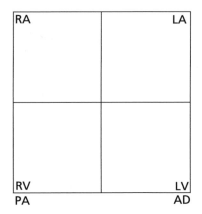

1. Mark the saturations in the boxes.

    (a) Ask:
    Are the saturations on the left greater than 90? Yes = normal.
    Are the saturations on the right less than 80? Yes = normal.
    Are they staying the same as the blood passes from one chamber to the next?

    (b) A step up on the right indicates a left-to-right shunt.

    (c) A step down on the left indicates a right-to-left shunt.

2. Now mark all the blood pressures in the boxes.

   (a) All the right sides should be lower than the left.

   (b) If they are equal at any level then there may be shunting.

   (c) If there is a step down across a valve then it is suggestive of stenosis.

   (d) This is especially true if you see a higher than expected pressure in the chamber before the step down; for example, in pulmonary stenosis this would be in the right ventricle.

Examples:

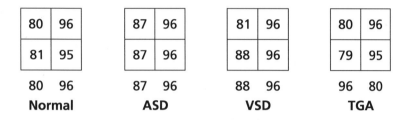

80	96
81	95

80   96
Normal

87	96
87	96

87   96
ASD

81	96
88	96

88   96
VSD

80	96
79	95

96   80
TGA

–/4	–/7
20/4	100/10

20/10   100/70
Normal

–/7	–/7
20/4	100/10

20/10   100/70
ASD

–/4	–/7
60/30	100/10

20/10   100/70
Pulmonary stenosis

2.6 You are reviewing a two-year-old with the following cardiac pressures. He is acyanotic:

	Pressure (mmHg)
RA	–/3
RV	50/20
Pulmonary	50/20
LA	–/7
LV	100/70
Aorta	100/70

(a) What is the diagnosis?
- (i)   ASD
- (ii) VSD
- (iii) PDA
- (iv) Normal
- (v)   Pulmonary stenosis

(b) What saturations would you expect in:
- (i)   RA?
- (ii) RV?

2.7 You see a three-week-old baby whom you suspect has cyanotic heart disease. These are the cardiac catheterization results:

	Saturation (%)
RA	80
RV	80
Pulmonary	95
LA	95
LV	95
Aortic	80

(a) Are you right?

(b) What is the diagnosis?
  (i) normal
  (ii) VSD
  (iii) tetralogy of Fallot
  (iv) TGA
  (v) PDA

2.8 A five-year-old child is seen by the cardiologist having been referred for a murmur that radiates to his back.

Cardiac catheterization shows:

	Pressure (mmHg)	Saturation (%)
RV	41/6	80
Left pulmonary	25/15	89
Aorta	98/53	99

(a) What is the diagnosis?
  (i) pulmonary stenosis
  (ii) left pulmonary stenosis
  (iii) coarctation
  (iv) right pulmonary stenosis
  (v) PDA

(b) What is the treatment of choice?
  (i) leave – stenosis will settle
  (ii) balloon dilatation
  (iii) coil device
  (iv) PDA ligation
  (v) open correction of coarctation

2.9 These are the cardiac catheterization pressures of a 13-year-old pre and post intervention:

	Pre Intervention	Post Intervention
Left ventricle	155/30	139/23
Ascending aorta	95/7	98/54
Descending aorta	109/63	

(a) What is the diagnosis?
  - (i)   aortic stenosis
  - (ii) coarctation
  - (iii) hypoplastic arch
  - (iv) PDA
  - (v)   corrected tetralogy of Fallot

(b) Give two ways he may have presented.

2.10 A six-month-old baby with known Fallot's is up for cardiac review. Pick two of the following which are most likely to be on the ECG:

  - (i)   RVH
  - (ii)   LVH
  - (iii) RAH
  - (iv)   RBBB
  - (v)   partial RBBB
  - (vi)   R axis deviation
  - (vii) L axis deviation
  - (viii) heart block

2.11 You are reviewing the ECG of a one-year-old baby. The rate is 76 and you are trying to work out the axis. Which of the following would stop that being possible?

  - (i)   partial RBBB
  - (ii) first-degree heart block
  - (iii) complete RBBB
  - (iv) intermittent ventricular ectopics
  - (v)   biventricular hypertrophy

2.12 A three-month-old is reviewed by the cardiologist. The echo confirms he has an ostium primum. Which of the following would you find on ECG (choose two)?

> (i)   RBBB
> (ii)   partial LBBB
> (iii) RVH
> (iv)   RAH
> (v)   L axis deviation
> (vi)   R axis deviation
> (vii) LBBB
> (viii) partial RBBB
> (ix)   LVH
> (x)   LAH

2.13 A three-month-old is referred to the regional cardiologist with a suspected VSD. Which of the following cardiac catheterizations would confirm your diagnosis?

	RA	RV	PA	LA	LV	A
(i)	60	70	69	96	96	96
(ii)	60	60	60	95	96	95
(iii)	80	80	80	96	96	96
(iv)	65	65	75	96	96	96
(v)	60	62	60	85	85	85

ANSWERS (2)

2.6 **(a)** (ii) (could be patent ductus arteriosus (PDA) but part **(b)** suggests VSD)

(b) (i) 80 (ii) 86
Comment: The pressure is increased in the right ventricle so in **(b)** show a step up here.

2.7 **(a)** Yes.

(b) (iv)
Comment: Be careful – at first glance the saturations look normal.

2.8 **(a)** (v)

(b) (iii)
Comment: The increase in both saturations and pressure shows a left-to-right shunt.

2.9 **(a)** (i)

(b) Incidental murmur or collapse.
Comment: This is caused by a drop in blood pressure across the valve.

2.10 (i) and (vi)
Comment: If in doubt write the four clinical points of Fallot's – RVH, overriding aorta, VSD and pulmonary stenosis – and think how they could affect the ECG.

2.11 (iii)
Comment: Complete right or left bundle branch block makes the axis impossible.

2.12 (v) and (viii)
Comment: Ostium Primum = left axis; ostium secundum = Right axis. There is one R in each.

2.13 (i)
Comment: Draw the boxes; if in doubt write the diagnosis for each. There is plenty of time.

ECGs

3.1 Comment on the axis of this ECG:

    (i)   normal
    (ii)   superior axis
   (iii) left axis
   (iv) right axis
    (v) cannot comment

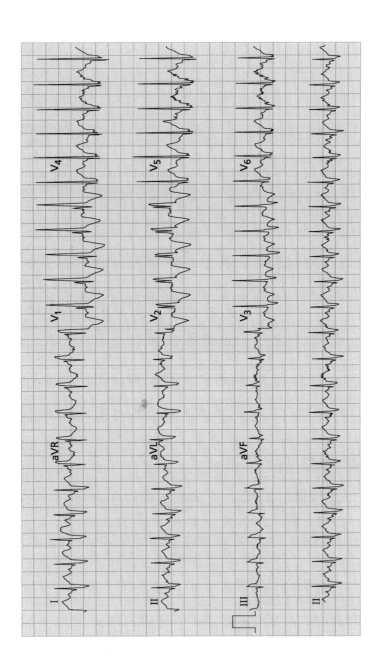

3.2 This is the ECG of a 14-year-old girl who had a Fontan operation for tricuspid atresia and pulmonary stenosis. Comment on the right atrium and ventricle:

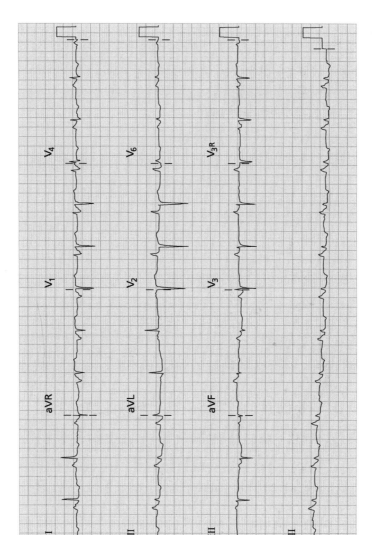

   (i)   normal atrium and ventricle
  (ii)   normal atrium and absent ventricle
 (iii)   enlarged atrium and absent ventricle
 (iv)   enlarged atrium and normal ventricle
  (v)   enlarged atrium and enlarged ventricle

3.3 This is the ECG of a five-year-old girl who was operated on for transposition. List three features on it that indicate right ventricular hypertrophy:

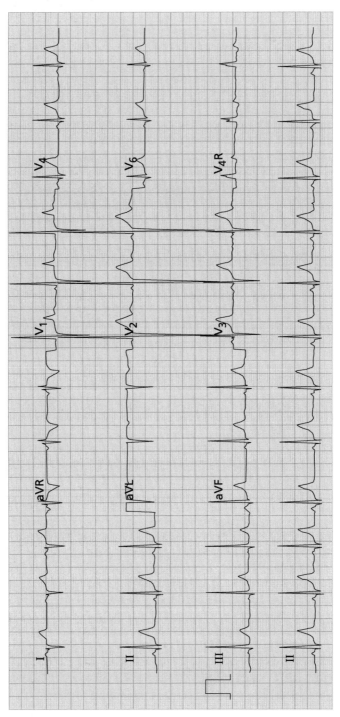

3.4 This 20-day-old baby with Down's syndrome has cyanosis.

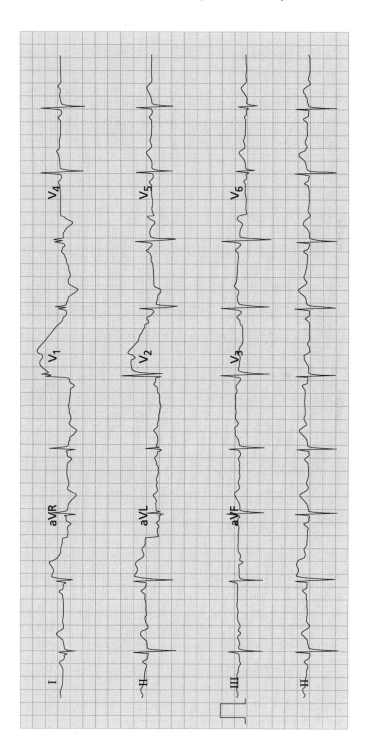

(a) Comment on the ECG:
- (i) complete RBBB
- (ii) partial RBBB with right axis deviation
- (iii) partial RBBB
- (iv) partial RBBB with left axis deviation
- (v) normal ECG

(b) What is the cause of the cyanosis?

3.1 (v)

Comment: Cannot comment as complete heart block. Look at V_1–M-wave; therefore RBBB (see hints).

3.2 (iii)

Comment: Peaked P-wave and V_3R is all negative.

3.3 Right axis.

Upright T-wave V_1 V_2.

Peaked R-wave V_1.

3.4 **(a)** (iv)

(b) Right to left shunt, through AVSD – secondary to pulmonary hypertension.

Comment: Associate the answer with the syndrome! It is not Eisenmenger's, because at this age it is caused by pulmonary hypertension and is reversible.

Helpful hints

HOW TO READ AN ECG

1. Look at the rhythm strip for:

   (a) Rate.
   (b) Rhythm.
   (c) Is there a P-wave for each QRS?

2. Look at leads V_1–V_6 to see where V_4R is. Look at the standardization mark to check millivoltage.

3. Look at the axis.
   Either:

   (a) I and aVF.

   Work out the number of positive or negative squares and then plot the axis.

   For example:

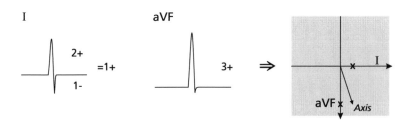

   Or:

(b) The axis is at right angles to the smallest most equiphasic lead. Then look at the lead at right angles; if it is positive the axis is towards it.

For example, if the equiphasic lead is aVf look at lead I:

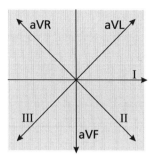

4. Look for bundle branch block (BBB). This is usually right BBB with M in V$_1$. Left BBB is exceptionally uncommon both in child and paediatric examinations (largely because it is not associated with congenital heart disease).

    Pnemonic: Marrow and William

    M M in lead V$_1$

    A

    R R for right

    R

    O

    W W in lead V$_6$

    W W in lead V$_1$

    I

    L L for left

    L

    I

    A

    M M in lead V$_6$

    NB:

    (a) Complete BBB (that is, wide QRS complex) means you cannot comment on the axis.

    (b) Partial BBB (that is, normal-width QRS complex) means you can comment on the axis.

    (c) RBBB means you cannot comment on right ventricular hypertrophy.

5. Look for atrial hypertrophy in leads II, V1.

   (a) P-wave too tall = right atrium.

   (b) P-wave bifid = left atrium.

6. Remember age dominance:

   For example, at birth right ventricle

   Then mixed dominance

   Progressing to left ventricle.

   (a) Right ventricle dominant   Mainly R-wave V_1

                                        Mainly S-wave V_6

   (b) Left ventricle dominant   Mainly S-wave V_1

                                        Mainly R-wave V_6

   Dominance usually changes from right to left in the first months.

7. Look for ventricular hypertrophy:

   (a) Right ventricular hypertrophy:

       R-wave > 20 mm V_1

       S-wave > 5 mm V_6

       Right axis deviation

       Positive T-wave V_1.

   (b) Left ventricular hypertrophy:

       S-wave > 20 mm V_1

       R-wave > 25 mm V_6.

   (c) Combined is a mixture of the above.

8. Look for a delta wave. This must be associated with a short P–R interval. (P–R is from start of P-wave until start of QRS complex. Normal 0.12 ms = 3 squares.) It may help to place a piece of paper along the R-wave.

    NB: This may be mistaken for BBB.

9. The T-wave should be negative from day 7 until 12 years in V_1.

10. Flat T = K^+ ↓   or = Ca^{2+} ↑

    Peaked T = K^+ ↑   or = Ca^{2+} ↓

    Now you have read the ECG, read the question and fit it together.

    For example:

    (a) Partial RBBB   = ASD

           Then right axis = secundum

           Left axis   = primum

           (Remember one R in each.)

    (b) Left ventricular hypertrophy.

    Think coarctation and aortic stenosis, for example.

3.5 This is the ECG of a 12-year-old girl who had a Fontan procedure for tricuspid atresia. There is no murmur and BP is 85/50.

What does the ECG show?

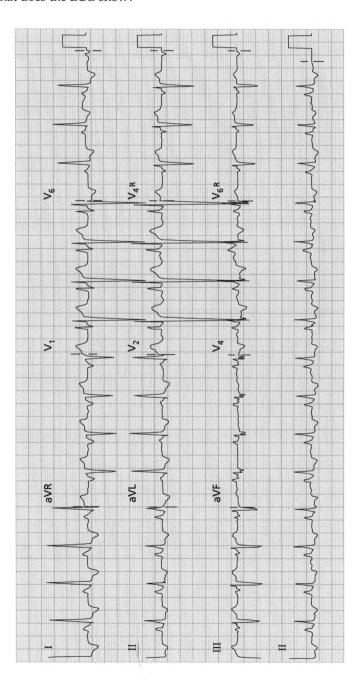

3.6 You have seen a three-month-old baby with the cardiologist. The baby has poor weight gain and feeding difficulty. The echocardiogram shows significant pulmonary artery branch stenosis.

(a) What is the likely diagnosis?
  (i) Down's syndrome
  (ii) cri du chat
  (iii) Prader–Willi syndrome
  (iv) Williams' syndrome
  (v) Angelman's syndrome

(b) How is this confirmed?

(c) What other blood test needs checking?

3.7 This is an ECG of a 16-year-old boy who is normally asymptomatic but was noted to have ectopics during surgery:

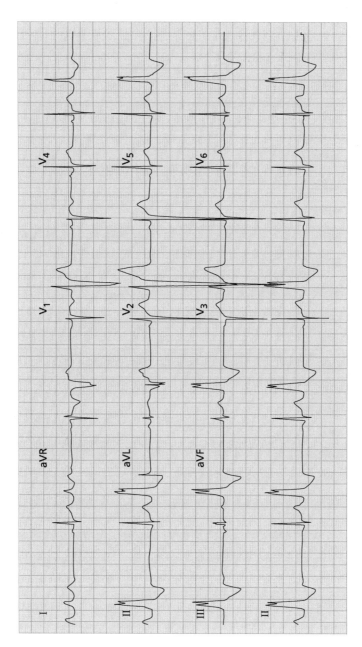

(a) What does the ECG show?

(b) Is he likely to need an operation?

(c) How might you confirm that they are benign?

3.8 You are reviewing a five-month-old baby with known pulmonary artery branch stenosis with the following ECG.

What features are notable on the ECG?

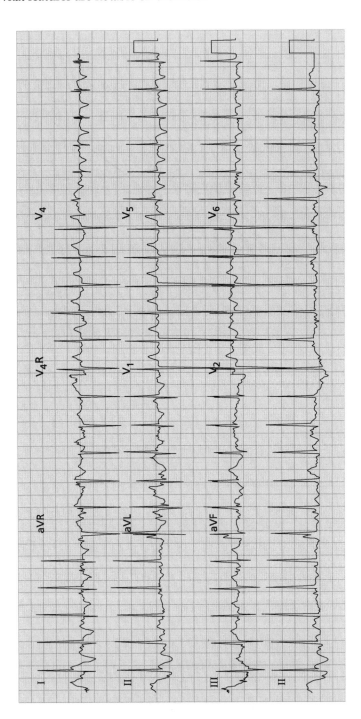

3.5   Right atrial hypertrophy.

Left axis deviation.

3.6   **(a)**   (iv)

(b)   FISH test: deletion long arm chromosome 7.

(c)   Calcium can be hypercalcaemic.
Comment: You can use initials but where possible write in full.

3.7   **(a)**   Bigemini with unifocal ventricular ectopics.

(b)   No.

(c)   They disappear with exercise.
Comment: Asymptomatic and normal complex in between.

3.8   Upright T-wave V_1.

Inverted T-wave V_6.
Comment: Look for the clue in the question – for example: pulmonary stenosis, therefore look at the right ventricle.

Audiometry

4.1 You are asked to see a five-year-old boy whose mother is worried that he watches television with the volume turned up too loud.

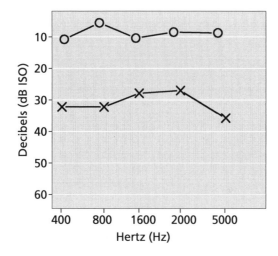

What is the diagnosis?

- (i) right conductive deafness
- (ii) left conductive deafness
- (iii) right and left conductive deafness
- (iv) right sensorineural deafness
- (v) left sensorineural deafness

4.2   You are asked to review the following Rinne and Weber results:

Right	Rinne positive
Left	Rinne negative
Weber	to the left

What would you expect the audiogram to show?

    (i)   normal right and left ear
   (ii)   normal left and conductive loss right
  (iii)   normal right and conductive loss left
  (iv)   normal right and sensorineural loss left
   (v)   normal left and sensorineural loss right

4.3 You are shown the following audiogram of a six-year-old who has a complication of a childhood illness:

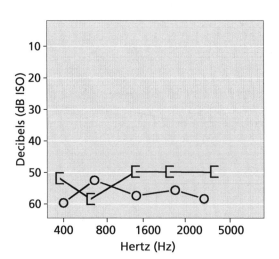

(a) What does it show?
    (i) left conductive loss
    (ii) bilateral conductive loss
    (iii) bilateral sensorineural loss
    (iv) left sensorineural loss
    (v) right sensorineural loss

(b) Name a possible childhood illness.

4.4 A four-year-old boy is tired during the day and dribbling a lot. He is developmentally normal.

(a) What two questions would you ask?

(b) Name two tests to confirm the diagnosis.

4.5 A child has sensorineural deafness on the left. What would be the results from Rinne and Weber tests?

	Rinne left	Rinne right	Weber
(i)	–ive	+ive	right
(ii)	–ive	–ive	right
(iii)	+ive	–ive	left
(iv)	+ive	+ive	central
(v)	–ive	–ive	left

4.6 These are the tympanogram results from a three-year-old boy.

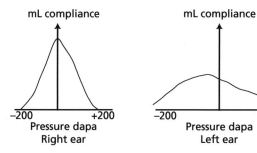

What diagnosis does it suggest?

   (i)   otitis media left
   (ii)   otitis media right
   (iii)   perforation left
   (iv)   poor seal on the left
   (v)   poor seal on the right

4.1 (ii)
Comments: Always make sure you indicate which ear. The hearing loss is less than 40 decibels, so is conductive.

4.2 (iii)

Normal right ear.
Comment: The ear that is Rinne negative is always the abnormal one.

4.3 **(a)** (v)

(b) Mumps or meningitis.

4.4 **(a)** Does he snore? Does he have pauses in his snoring?

(b) Overnight saturations. Arterial blood gas while asleep.
Comment: Diagnosis is usually made on history.

4.5 (i)

4.6 (i)
Comment: Left tympanogram flattened and shifted to the left.

Helpful hints

AUDIOMETRY

1. Which ear? This is easily remembered by Right O (chaps), and therefore X is left.

2. Normal hearing is from 0 → −20.

3. Conductive hearing loss from −20 → −40.

4. Sensorineural loss is from −40+.

5. If the examiners give you a conductive hearing loss of greater than −40 then they will also give bone conduction, which will be a lot better.

6. If the examiners give you a sensorineural hearing loss of less than −40 then they will show bone conduction at a similar level.

Examples

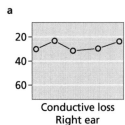

a

Conductive loss
Right ear

b

Sensorineural
Left ear

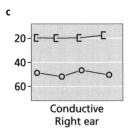

c

Conductive
Right ear

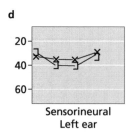

d

Sensorineural
Left ear

The Rinne test compares air and bone conduction for one ear, and is performed by putting the tuning fork near the ear until it cannot be heard, then putting it on the mastoid process. If it is audible again then it is Rinne negative.

The Weber test compares the bone conduction of both ears. The tuning fork is placed in the centre of the forehead.

1. The ear that is Rinne negative is always the abnormal one.

2. If the Weber test is towards the abnormal ear it is conductive hearing loss.

3. If the Weber test is away from that ear it is sensorineural hearing loss.

4. If both Rinne tests are negative then:

    (a) Weber central means that both ears have either sensorineural or conductive loss.

    (b) Weber towards one ear means that ear has conductive loss and the other ear sensorineural loss.

4.7 This is the audiogram of a five-year-old girl:

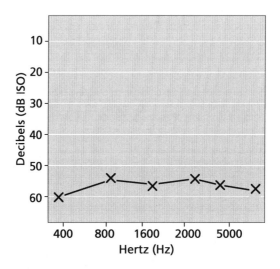

(a) Which ear is it?

(b) Add:
  (i) bone conduction for sensorineural deafness
  (ii) bone conduction for conductive deafness

4.8 These are the tympanograms of a two-year-old boy:

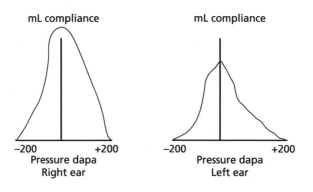

If the left ear is normal, what would you expect to see in the right ear on examination?

4.9 This is the hearing test of a six-year-old boy with Down's syndrome:

Right	Rinne negative
Left	Rinne negative
Weber	central

(a) What is the differential diagnosis?

(b) Which diagnosis is more likely?

4.10 This is an audiogram of a three-year-old referred to an ENT surgeon:

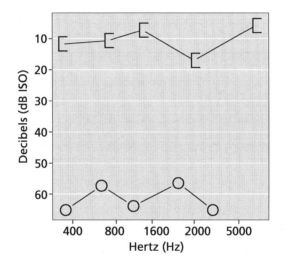

(a) What does it show?
- (i) severe sensorineural loss – right
- (ii) moderate sensorineural loss – left
- (iii) severe conductive loss – left
- (iv) severe conductive loss – right
- (v) moderate conductive loss – right

(b) Does he need an operation?

4.7 **(a)** The left ear.

(b)

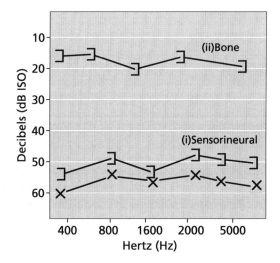

4.8 The right ear may be normal, but may have a thin eardrum (hypermobile) or ossicular discontinuity.

4.9 **(a)** Bilateral conductive or sensorineural hearing loss.

(b) Conductive.
Comment: Conductive hearing loss is more common in Down's syndrome babies, but also in any child with a facial problem such as cleft palate or snoring.

4.10 **(a)** (iv)

(b) Yes.

Neurology

5

QUESTIONS (1)

5.1 A 13-year-old boy is admitted with his second generalized tonic–clonic seizure, but on closer questioning is said to be quite 'jumpy' in the mornings, such that he tends to spill drinks at breakfast and drop his pen at school. The EEG findings are shown below.

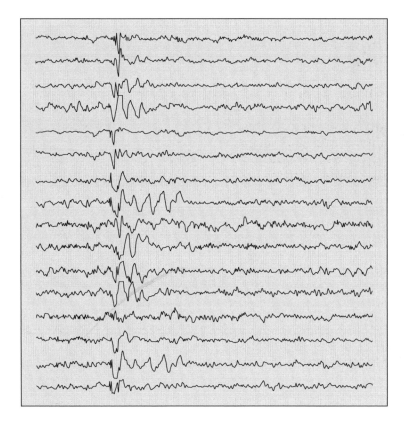

(a) Describe the EEG:
  (i)   generalized regular spike wave complex
  (ii) burst suppression
  (iii) generalized irregular spike wave complex
  (iv) left-sided irregular spike wave complex
  (v)   generalized spike discharge

(b) What is the diagnosis?
  (i)   juvenile myoclonic epilepsy
  (ii) benign Rolandic epilepsy
  (iii) absence epilepsy
  (iv) partial epilepsy
  (v)   complex partial epilepsy

5.2 At six days old, a baby girl developed myoclonic and tonic seizures, unresponsive to standard anti-epilepsy drugs. Daily seizures continued unabated, and the EEG at four weeks of age is shown:

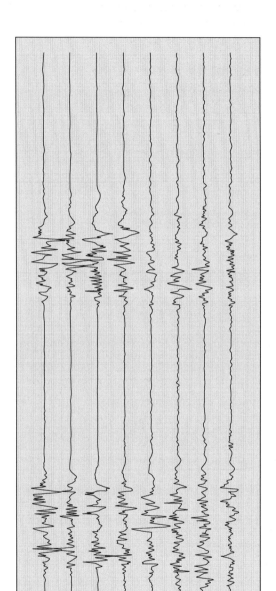

(a) Describe the EEG pattern:
- (i) generalized irregular spike wave pattern
- (ii) hypsarrhythmia
- (iii) temporal spike discharges
- (iv) normal
- (v) burst suppression pattern

(b) Suggest a likely diagnosis.

5.3 A seven-year-old girl was referred because of concerns about lapses in concentration and deterioration in school work:

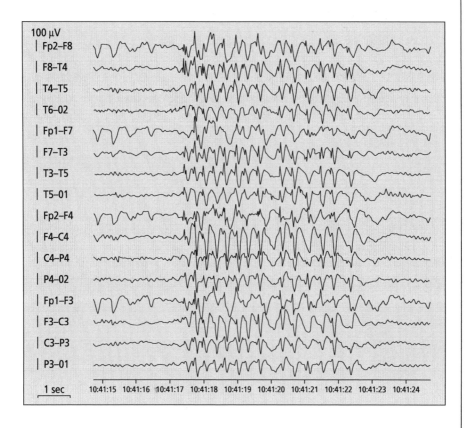

(a) What does the EEG demonstrate?
- (i) generalized 3 per second spike and wave discharge
- (ii) burst suppression pattern
- (iii) hypsarrhythmia
- (iv) normal
- (v) generalized spike discharges

(b) What practical manoeuvre may help with the diagnosis in clinic?

(c) What is the diagnosis?

5.4 An eight-month-old infant, admitted with crying episodes, is noted to have intermittent abnormal movements causing distress:

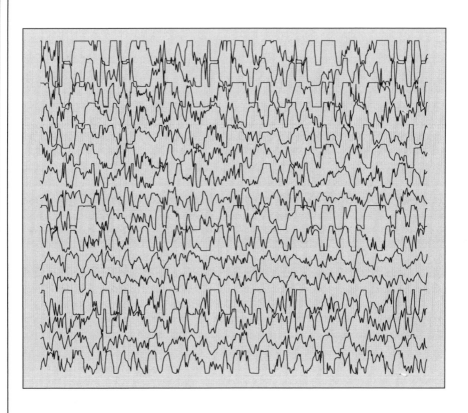

(a) What does his EEG show?
   (i) normal
   (ii) generalized spike discharges
   (iii) hypsarrhythmia
   (iv) burst suppression pattern
   (v) temporal spike discharges

(b) What is the diagnosis?
   (i) neonatal myoclonic epilepsy
   (ii) HIE grade III
   (iii) normal
   (iv) infantile spasms
   (v) drug withdrawal

5.5 An 11-year-old girl presented with a three-month history of episodic staring lasting two minutes, accompanied by excessive swallowing and occasional inappropriate laughter:

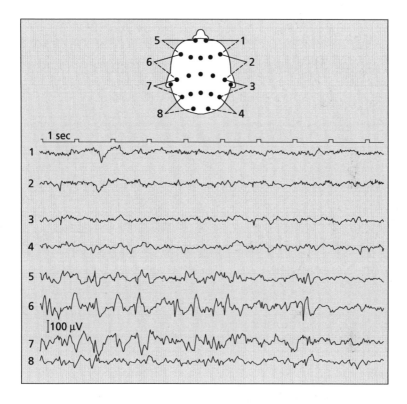

(a) Describe the EEG findings.
- (i) left temporal spike discharge
- (ii) right temporal spike discharge
- (iii) left parietal spike discharge
- (iv) right parietal spike discharge
- (v) left occipital spike discharge

(b) What is the diagnosis?

(c) What is the most appropriate next investigation?

5.1 **(a)** (iii)

(b) (i)
Comment: History and age are important: 'jumpy' with spills in the morning (or when tired) = myoclonic seizures; often presents as first/second generalized tonic–clonic seizure; EEG generalized (across whole montage) with short-lived spike-wave discharge.

5.2 **(a)** (v)

(b) Severe early neonatal myoclonic epilepsy.
Comment: History, age, very early onset and progressive (malignant). EEG shows bursts of abnormal chaotic activity on a very flat virtually iso-electric background – very ominous and typical of burst suppression.

5.3 **(a)** (i)

(b) Hyperventilation.

(c) Childhood onset typical of absence epilepsy.

Comment:

– The history may not make specific reference to absences.

– Watch out for the same question with normal EEG (the diagnosis may then be attentional/learning difficulties).

– Age is important for precise diagnosis (childhood onset, juvenile onset etc.)

– Do not use the term petit mal.

– Slower frequency may indicate atypical absence epilepsy.

– Beware hyperventilation indicator on montage.

This is a blueprint (diagnostic) EEG.

5.4 **(a)** (iii)

(b) (iv)

Comment: History – a common presentation masquerading as colic. It could be West's syndrome, but there is no specific mention of developmental delay at presentation. The underlying diagnosis (for example, tuberous sclerosis) cannot be determined by EEG alone. Blueprint EEG diagnostic when present – chaotic disorganized background with multifocal high-amplitude spikes and slow waves.

5.5 **(a)** (i)

(b) Complex partial seizures.

(c) MRI of the brain.

Comment: History – episodes too long for typical absence, and associated with unusual mannerisms, suggest complex partial seizures (formerly known as temporal lobe epilepsy). EEG – focal spike discharges in leads 6 and 7 (left temporal region). MRI is now the first-choice investigation for looking at temporal lobes in detail.

Helpful hints

THE EEG

1. Read the history carefully as this can give the diagnosis before looking at the EEG.

2. EEG abnormalities are likely to be obvious or 'blueprint'/diagnostic.

3. Montage (that is, orientation of leads):

   - Left is left and right is right as you look at the montage.
   - Labelling may vary but should always allow you to match up the labels on the montage with the corresponding leads on the EEG (and hence identify relevant area of the brain).
   - Ignore the montage if the abnormality is apparent across all leads (that is, generalized).
   - If there is no montage in the examination the EEG is very likely to show a generalized abnormality.

4. Basic principles:

   - Is the abnormality across all leads? If so, this is a generalized epilepsy.
   - Is the abnormality across the leads of one side/one or two leads only? If so, this is a partial/focal epilepsy.
   - Is the abnormality paroxysmal, for example spike-wave discharges/spike discharges?
   - Is the abnormality periodic, for example burst suppression or SSPE?
   - Is the abnormality continuous, for example hypsarrhythmia or status epilepticus?
   - Is the abnormality rhythmic or disorganized/chaotic?

5. Look for:

   (a) Second (time-scale) marker to identify frequency (for instance, 3 per second spike-wave discharge).

   (b) Photic stimulation marker – may precede photo-paroxysmal response.

   (c) Hyperventilation marker – may precede 3 per second spike-wave discharges.

   (d) ECG trace (at the bottom of the EEG recording). This may identify alternative (for example, cardiac) cause for collapse.

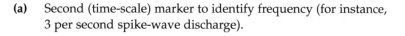

5.6 A 14-year-old girl with moderate learning difficulties and myoclonic epilepsy presented with a 24-hour history of unresponsiveness, staring and fumbling with her clothes. The EEG shown is representative of the whole 20-minute EEG recording:

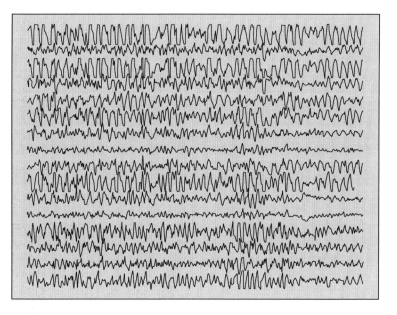

(a) What is the diagnosis?
  (i) encephalopathy
  (ii) complex partial status epilepticus
  (iii) Lennox–Gastaut syndrome
  (iv) subacute sclerosing panencephalitis
  (v) benign

(b) What would be your immediate management?

5.7 A 10-year-old boy, initially referred to the child psychiatrist with a behavioural disorder, has shown a progressive deterioration in written work over the last six months at school. More recently he has fallen over a number of times, appearing to lose his balance:

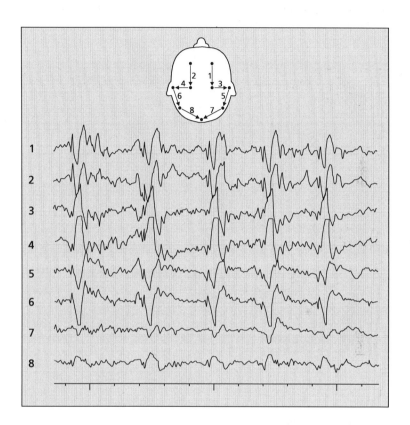

(a) What does his EEG show?
  (i)   normal
  (ii)   hypsarrhythmia
  (iii) burst suppression wave
  (iv)   large-amplitude periodic slow-wave complexes
  (v)   spike waves discharge

(b) What is the diagnosis?
  (i)   encephalopathy
  (ii)   complex partial status epilepticus
  (iii) Lennox–Gastaut syndrome
  (iv)   subacute sclerosing panencephalitis
  (v)   benign Rolandic

5.8 An eight-year-old boy presents in the early hours of the morning, following his first generalized tonic–clonic seizure. On closer questioning, it is found that he has experienced frequent episodes of unilateral facial paraesthesia for four months, followed by choking sensations and twitching of the lips and cheek. These occur on awakening, and he is unable to communicate during such episodes:

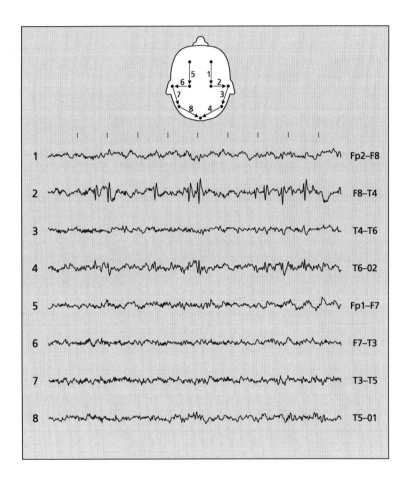

(a) What does his EEG demonstrate?

    (i)   unilateral right sided centro-temporal spike waves

    (ii)   unilateral left sided centro-temporal spike waves

    (iii) bilateral centro-temporal spike waves

    (iv) bilateral centro-temporal spikes

    (v)   normal

(b) What is the diagnosis?
- (i) encephalopathy
- (ii) complex partial status epilepticus
- (iii) Lennox–Gastaut syndrome
- (iv) subacute sclerosing panencephalitis
- (v) benign Rolandic

5.9 A seven-year-old boy with severe learning difficulties was diagnosed with West's syndrome at six months of age, and continues to experience frequent multiple seizure types (including tonic, atonic and myoclonic seizures):

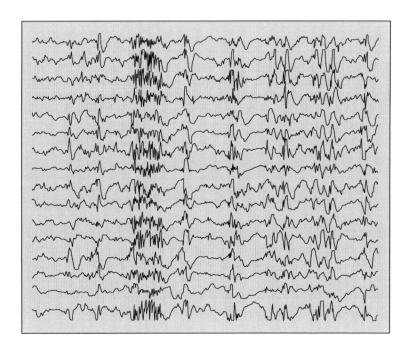

(a) Describe his EEG:
- (i)   normal
- (ii)   generalized multiple discharges of spike-wave and poly-spike complexes
- (iii) hypsarrhythmia
- (iv)   burst suppression
- (v)   generalized spike-wave complexes

(b) What is the diagnosis?
- (i)   encephalopathy
- (ii)   complex partial status epilepticus
- (iii) Lennox–Gastaut syndrome
- (iv)   subacute sclerosing panencephalitis
- (v)   benign Rolandic

5.10 A teenage boy has juvenile myoclonic epilepsy:

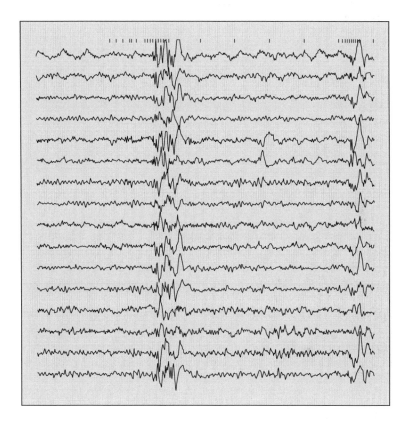

(a) What has the technician done?
  (i)   hyperventilation
  (ii) sleep-deprived EEG
  (iii) got the child to talk
  (iv) nothing
  (v)   photostimulation

(b) What might the technician have witnessed during this period of the recording?

5.6 **(a)** (ii)

(b) Intravenous bolus of diazepam.
Comment: The history is very suggestive of complex partial/atypical absence/non-convulsive status epilepticus. EEG shows a virtually continuous slow wave activity across all leads, and throughout the whole of the recording. Treatment is with intravenous benzodiazepine rather than rectal (because of 24-hour history). May need infusion; this is often undertaken 'under EEG control', but this is not essential and will usually see the patient 'wake up' following/during administration.

5.7 **(a)** (iv)

(b) (iv)
Comment: Look at the history and age (in fact 10 years is quite young for SSPE). Patients are often referred as having behavioural/psychiatric problems. There is progressive neurological regression including ataxia. EEG shows typical periodic appearance across all leads.

5.8 **(a)** (i)

(b) (v)
Comment: The history and age are important. Typical presentation in early hours of the morning (usually during sleep); typical history of partial sensory motor seizures (involving face, plus or minus upper limb). Beware, as this often presents as apparent first generalized tonic–clonic seizure (but is a partial epilepsy). Alternative label/diagnosis is 'benign partial epilepsy of childhood with centro-temporal (Rolandic) spikes'. Blueprint EEG and diagnostic.

5.9 **(a)** (ii)

(b) (iii)
Comment: History – Important cause of developmental arrest – intractable multiple seizure types are often resistant to standard anti-epileptic drugs. Age at presentation is important. Previous history of West's syndrome is common. EEG is not as chaotic as hypsarrhythmia – multiple spikes and poly-spikes are typical.

5.10 **(a)** (v)

(b) Myoclonic jerk.
Comment: Look at the EEG photic stimulation 'markers'. It would be reasonable to suggest myoclonic jerk, absence or eyelid flickering as a clinical (photo-convulsive) response. May have similar EEG photo-paroxysmal response without any clinical change.

Genetics

QUESTIONS (1)

6.1 You are seeing patients (a) and (b) below who show you the following family tree:

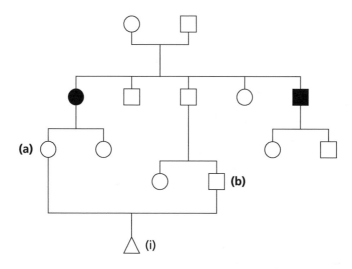

(a) What is the mode of inheritance?
- (i) autosomal recessive
- (ii) autosomal dominant
- (iii) X-linked recessive
- (iv) X-linked dominant
- (v) mitochondrial

(b) If you were seeing (a) and (b) antenatally, what is the chance of (a) having the condition?
- (i) 1/8
- (ii) 1/10
- (iii) 1/12
- (iv) 1/14
- (v) 1/16

6.2 The following family history has been worked out:

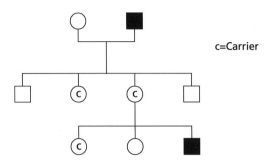

c=Carrier

What is the mode of inheritance?

  (i)   autosomal recessive
  (ii) autosomal dominant
  (iii) X-linked recessive
  (iv) X-linked dominant
  (v)   mitochondrial

6.3 A baby is born with a cleft palate and found to have a heart murmur. This is shown to be tetralogy of Fallot.

(a) What is the likely diagnosis?
  (i)   Down's syndrome
  (ii) Crouzon's syndrome
  (iii) Di George's syndrome
  (iv) Patau's syndrome
  (v)   Edwards' syndrome

(b) Name a confirmatory test.

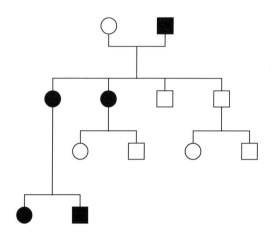

What is the mode of inheritance?

    (i)   autosomal recessive
    (ii)   autosomal dominant
   (iii)   X-linked recessive
   (iv)   X-linked dominant
    (v)   mitochondrial

6.5 The karyotype is 46 XY − 14 + t (14q 21q).

Describe the above.

6.6 A girl is admitted, drowsy, having had a history of a viral illness. There is a family history of SIDS and her mother has an increased orotic acid.

(a) What is the likely diagnosis?

(b) What is its mode of inheritance?
    (i)   autosomal recessive
    (ii)   autosomal dominant
   (iii)   X-linked recessive
   (iv)   X-linked dominant
    (v)   mitochondrial

(c) How will you confirm the diagnosis?

6.1 **(a)** (i)

(b) (iii)
Comment:

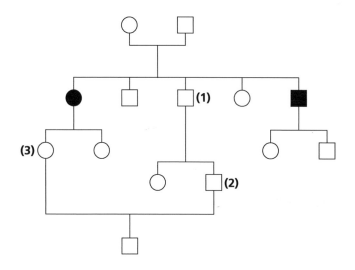

Look at one generation at a time.

For example (1) =

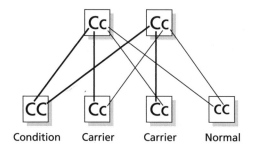

Cc	Cc
CC	Cc	Cc	CC
Condition	Carrier	Carrier	Normal

As we already know that (1) has not got the condition, ⅔ are carriers.

Then (2) = ½ because we assume that (1) marries a non-carrier.
(3) Again, assuming that the father is a non-carrier then the mother must pass the affected gene on.

6.2 (iii)
Comment: The father passes it to all his daughters, but they are only carriers, and none of his sons. The mother can make daughters carriers and affect sons.

6.3 **(a)** (iii)

(b) FISH assay looking at chromosome 22.
Comment: This is an example of best fitting a syndrome to a set of clinical features.

6.4 (iv)
Comment: Always look to see who can inherit from whom. It could be autosomal dominant but the tree shows two sons not getting it from their father.

6.5 Male unbalanced Robertsonian 14, 21 translocation.
Comment: Do not forget to mention the sex of the fetus.

6.6 **(a)** Ornithine carbamyl transferase deficiency.

(b) (iii)

(c) Urinary orotic acid levels.

Helpful hints

GENETICS

1. Autosomal dominant + recessive can go from mother and father to sons and daughters.

2. Autosomal recessive usually results from relations marrying.

3. X-linked recessive: mothers can only give it to sons and daughters have 50/50 chance of carriage.

4. X-linked recessive: fathers cannot give it to sons and all daughters carry it.

5. X-linked dominant: mothers may give it to sons or daughters (50/50).

6. X-linked dominant: fathers cannot give it to sons and give it to all daughters.

7. Do not forget the occasional mitochondrial inheritance which comes only from mothers.

6.7 A 19-year-old girl asks to see you. Her brother has cystic fibrosis.

What is the approximate risk of her child having it?

   (i)   1 in 100
   (ii) 1 in 120
   (iii) 1 in 160
   (iv) 1 in 200
   (v)   1 in 360

6.8 You are asked to see a four-month-old girl who has lines of warts on her limbs. She was noted to have some vesicles in the first few days of life.

(a) What is the diagnosis?

(b) What is the mode of inheritance?
   (i)   autosomal recessive
   (ii) autosomal dominant
   (iii) X-linked recessive
   (iv) X-linked dominant
   (v)   mitochondrial

6.9 You are asked to see a 13-year-old girl because of her short stature. She has not entered puberty. Her LH/FSH are greatly raised.

(a) What is the diagnosis?

(b) How would you confirm this?

6.10

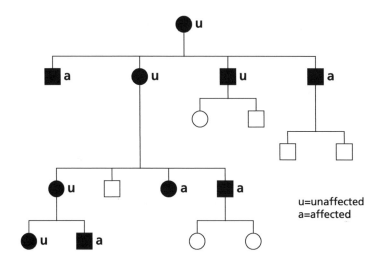

u=unaffected
a=affected

If this is not X-linked, what is the mode of inheritance?
- (i)   autosomal recessive
- (ii) autosomal dominant
- (iii) X-linked recessive
- (iv) X-linked dominant
- (v)   mitochondrial

6.11 You are reviewing a one-year-old child known to be hypertensive (127/65). He has the following investigation results:

Extra part of chromosome 15 on 19

Peripheral pulmonary branch stenosis

Horseshoe kidney – bilateral patchy uptake left 55% and right 45%.

(a) Why is he hypertensive?
- (i)   chromosome anomaly
- (ii) cardiac lesion
- (iii) renal scar
- (iv) horseshoe kidney
- (v)   Essential hypertension

(b) Name a possible treatment.

6.12 You are reviewing a nine-year-old boy with learning difficulties who you last saw six months ago. He appears to have a prominent jaw and large, prominent ears. You also note some stereotype behaviour. You feel he has fragile X and chromosomal analysis confirms this. In what range would you expect the mother's repeat frequency to be?

    (i)   <10
   (ii)   10–50
  (iii) 50–200
  (iv) 200–500
   (v) 500–1000

6.13 A couple come to you for genetic counselling. Their first child was a late miscarriage. Chromosome analysis showed Down's syndrome caused by translocation. This leads you to check the parents' chromosomes.

(a) If the mother is a carrier the recurrence risk is:
    (i)   1–3%
   (ii)   3–6%
  (iii) 6–10%
  (iv) 10–20%
   (v) 20–50%

(b) If the father is a carrier the recurrence risk is:
    (i)   1–3%
   (ii)   3–6%
  (iii) 6–10%
  (iv) 10–20%
   (v) 20–50%

6.14 A family tree is shown below:

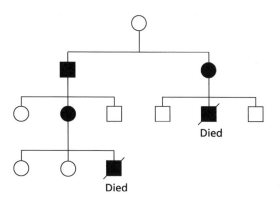

The pattern of inheritance is:

   (i)   autosomal recessive
  (ii)   autosomal dominant
 (iii) X-linked recessive
 (iv) mitochondrial
  (v)   X-linked dominant

6.7 $\frac{2}{3} \times \frac{1}{4} \times \frac{1}{20} = \frac{1}{120} = $ (ii)

$\frac{2}{3}$ = her chance of being a carrier.

$\frac{1}{4}$ = chance of offspring having cystic fibrosis if both parents have it.

$\frac{1}{20}$ = carrier rate (between $\frac{1}{20}$ and $\frac{1}{25}$).

6.8 **(a)** Incontinentia pigmenti.

(b) (iv)
Comment: May also be presented as male deaths.

6.9 **(a)** Turner's syndrome.

(b) Chromosomes looking for 45X0.

6.10 (v)
Comment: Inheritance is only passed down the female line but to either sex.

6.11 **(a)** (iii)

(b) ACE inhibitor.

6.12 (iii)

6.13 **(a)** (iv)

(b) (i)

6.14 (v)
Comment: You are not being asked to show your knowledge of the chromosomal diagnosis.

Statistics

7

7.1 A trial of a new test gives the following results:

	Has disease	Does not have disease
Positive	90	10
Negative	10	90

(a) What is the sensitivity?
- (i) 10%
- (ii) 90%
- (iii) 500%
- (iv) 100%
- (v) 5%

(b) What is the specificity?
- (i) 10%
- (ii) 90%
- (iii) 50%
- (iv) 100%
- (v) 5%

7.2 On auditing urine results you find the following:

	Pure growth organism	Multiple growth
>50 WBC	95	15
<50 WBC	10	200

(a) What is the positive predictive value?
  (i) 95/105
  (ii) 95/110
  (iii) 95/210
  (iv) 95/200
  (v) 95/320

(b) What is the negative predictive value?
  (i) 10/210
  (ii) 200/215
  (iii) 200/210
  (iv) 10/105
  (v) 10/320

7.1 **(a)** (ii)

    (b) (ii)

7.2 **(a)** (ii)

    (b) (iii)

Helpful hints

2 × 2 CHARTS

Sensitivity = the proportion of people with the condition that the test picks up.

Specificity = the proportion of people without the condition that have a negative test.

Positive predictive value = the chance that someone has the condition if the test is positive.

Negative predictive value = the chance that someone does not have the condition if the test is negative.

For example:

Sensitivity	=	$\dfrac{a}{a+c}$
Specificity	=	$\dfrac{d}{d+b}$
Positive predictive value	=	$\dfrac{a}{a+b}$
Negative predictive value	=	$\dfrac{d}{d+c}$

	Have condition	Do not have condition
Positive test	a	b
Negative test	c	d

Comment: Make sure the chart is correctly oriented.

7.3 A test has a positive predictive value of 90 and a negative predictive value of 95. Draw an appropriate 2 × 2 table.

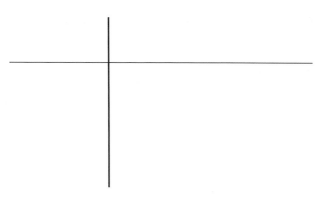

7.4 List five of the criteria for a screening programme.

7.3

	Have condition	Do not have condition
Positive	90	10
Negative	5	95

7.4   The condition is a serious one.

An acceptable test can pick up the condition before it is clinically detectable.

The disease course can be altered by early detection.

The test is highly sensitive and specific.

The programme is cost effective.

Electrolytes

QUESTIONS (1)

8.1 The following blood results were obtained from an 18-month-old failing to thrive:

Sodium	127 mmol/L
Potassium	2.6 mmol/L
Chloride	80 mmol/L

(a) What is the most likely diagnosis?
- (i) salt-losing congenital adrenal hyperplasia
- (ii) salt poisoning
- (iii) Bartter's syndrome
- (iv) pseudo-Bartter's syndrome
- (v) Addison's disease

(b) What is the pathophysiology?

PASS

8.2 The following results occurred in a three-day-old 26-week gestation neonate while on a radiant warmer:

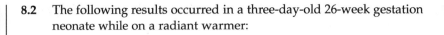

Sodium	147 mmol/L
Potassium	4.3 mmol/L
Urea	6.0 mmol/L
Creatinine	97 µmol/L

(a) What is the diagnosis?
  (i) normal
  (ii) inappropriate ADH
  (iii) diabetes insipidus
  (iv) sodium overload
  (v) dehydration

(b) Give two management strategies.

8.3 The following blood results were obtained on an ill six-year-old:

Sodium	135 mmol/L
Potassium	4.6 mmol/L
Urea	10.0 mmol/L
Osmolality	310 mOsm/kg

(a) What blood result is missing?

(b) Approximately what should the result be?
  (i) 5
  (ii) 10
  (iii) 15
  (iv) 20
  (v) 25

8.4 A 10-year-old child with diabetes is admitted semi-conscious. Urgent blood results are as follows:

Blood glucose	40+ mmol/L
Osmolality	350 mOsm/kg
pH	7.26

What is the diagnosis?
- (i) ketotic hyperglycaemia coma
- (ii) non-ketotic hyperglycaemia coma
- (iii) ketotic hyperosmolar coma
- (iv) non-ketotic hyperosmolar coma
- (v) drug overdose

8.1 **(a)** (iii)

(b) Vascular unresponsiveness to angiotensin; renal loss of chloride.
Comment: You need to always try to make the data fit the answer. In this case there is a low chloride; it may also give the pH. In Bartter's syndrome the pH shows an alkalosis; Pseudo-Bartter's syndrome may produce similar results but there is not enough information.

8.2 **(a)** (v)

(b) Place in a humidified incubator and increase the fluids.
Comment: Always put answers in order of importance as they may include things like 'recheck electrolytes later, cover with bubble sheet', and so on.

8.3 **(a)** Blood glucose.

(b) (iv)
Comment: Whenever osmolality is mentioned, work out approximately what it should be, for example 2 × [Na + K] + urea + glucose – often one is missing in the question.

8.4 (iv)
Comment: The high glucose would be appropriate for diabetic ketoacidosis (DKA) but you would expect a low pH if the patient was semi-conscious.

Helpful hints

ELECTROLYTE AND DEXTROSE SOLUTIONS

1. Dextrose as mg/kg/h

$$= \frac{10 \times \% \text{ dextrose} \times \text{ml/h}}{\text{wt} \times 60}$$

For example, 1 kg neonate on 7.5% dextrose at 120 ml/kg/day

$$= \frac{10 \times 7.5 \times {}^{120}\!/_{24}}{60}$$

$$\text{mg/kg/h} = \frac{10 \times 7.5 \times 5}{60} = \frac{37.5}{6} = 6.25$$

Normal is 5 mg/kg/h. There is a need to investigate only if low BM and >12 mg/kg/h.

2. Sodium: formula to work out deficit:

$0.6 \times \text{deficit} \times \text{wt in mmol/L}$

Be careful as dextrose is usually expressed in mg whereas everything else is in mmol.

3. 0.18% = 30 mmol/L

   0.9% = 150 mmol/L

   Note that 30% is usually easier to remember per millilitre

   = 5 mmol/ml

   Examples

   (a) 12 kg child with sodium 115 mmol/L

   Normal 135 mmol/L $\Rightarrow$ deficit = $(135 - 115) \times 0.6 \times 12 = 144$ mmol

   (b) Neonate on 1 ml/h of 0.45% saline

   150 ml/kg/day of dextrose 10% + 0.18% saline

   Is this neonate getting enough sodium?

   (They usually need 4 mmol/kg/day)

   Assume 1 kg

   $$\Rightarrow \frac{(24 \times 75)}{1000} + \frac{(150 \times 30)}{1000} = 6.3 \text{ mmol/kg/day}$$

4. Potassium: 10 mmol/500 ml = 0.15% KCl.

8.5 A child has a sodium of 118 mmol/L. The child weighs 20 kg and you want to increase his sodium to 135 mmol/L.

What is the deficit?
- (i) 104
- (ii) 154
- (iii) 204
- (iv) 254
- (v) 304

8.6 A seven-day-old neonate who is known to have septicaemia has the following results from his arterial line:

Sodium	135 mmol/L
Potassium	8.4 mmol/L
Urea	12.4 mmol/L
Creatinine	165 μmol/L

(a) What is the most likely cause of his high potassium?
- (i) renal failure
- (ii) inappropriate TPN
- (iii) inappropriate ADH secretion
- (iv) pre-renal failure
- (v) haemolysis

(b) List three treatment options to bring it down.

8.7 A four-day-old 28-week gestation neonate had a blood sugar reading of 1.6 mmol/L and this was only stabilized on 150 ml/kg/day of 10% dextrose.

(a) Does this warrant further investigation?

(b) Justify your answer.

8.8 You are asked to review a 29-week-gestation neonate who is one day old with poor urine output. The following results are available:

Hb	14.3 g/dL
WBC	3.5×10^9/L
Platelets	139×10^9/L
Sodium	127 mmol/L
Potassium	3.3 mmol/L

(a) What is the most likely diagnosis and cause?
  (i) fluid overload
  (ii) inappropriate ADH
  (iii) inappropriate TPN
  (iv) Bartter's syndrome
  (v) pseudo-Bartter's syndrome

(b) What fluid management is appropriate?

8.9 A 1 kg baby is receiving the following i.v. fluids:

UAC 0.45% NaCl 1 ml/h

Peripheral line 200 ml/kg/day of dextrose 10% + 0.18% NaCl

How many mmol/kg of sodium is this baby on?

  (i) 5.8
  (ii) 8.8
  (iii) 9.8
  (iv) 6.8
  (v) 7.8

8.5 (iii) $(135 - 118) \times 0.6 \times 20 = 204$ mmol
Comment: See hints.

8.6 **(a)** (iv)

(b) Fluid bolus; intravenous B dextrose and insulin; intravenous salbutamol.
Comment: Try to expand renal failure to fit with the history given.

8.7 **(a)** No.

(b)

$$\frac{\cancel{10} \times \cancel{10}^{\,5} \times \dfrac{\cancel{150}^{\;2}}{24}}{\underset{\cancel{3}\;\;1}{60}} = 10 \text{ mg/kg/h}$$

Do not investigate until >12 mg/kg/h.
Comment: Write down the calculation, then look at the answers.

8.8 **(a)** (ii)

(b) Fluid restriction.
Comment: Poor urine output is often because neonates are dehydrated, but here the sodium is low.

Umbilical artery catheter (UAC) 24 ml/day

0.45% NaCl = 75 mmol/L

$$\frac{\overset{3}{\cancel{24}}}{\underset{5}{\cancel{1000}}} \times \overset{3}{\cancel{75}} = \frac{9}{5} \text{ mmol}$$

Peripheral line 150 ml/day

0.18% = 30 mmol/L

$$\frac{\cancel{200}}{\cancel{1000}} \times 3\cancel{0} = 6 \text{ mmol}$$

Total = 7.8 mmol

Emergency medicine

QUESTIONS (1)

9.1 You are crash called to a two-year-old in A&E who is unresponsive to initial attempts to resuscitate.

    (a) How much would you expect him to weigh?
        (i)   8 kg
        (ii)   10 kg
        (iii) 12 kg
        (iv) 14 kg
        (v)   16 kg

    (b) What is an appropriate dose of adrenaline if administered via the endotracheal tube?
        (i)   0.8 ml of 1 in 1000
        (ii)   1 ml of 1 in 10 000
        (iii) 1.2 ml of 1 in 1000
        (iv) 0.8 ml of 1 in 10 000
        (v)   1.4 ml of 1 in 1000

9.2 A five-year-old child in intensive care is intubated with intravenous access, but has a cardiac arrest.

    (a) What are the first two things to do?

    (b) What are the first and subsequent doses of intravenous adrenaline?

9.3 A three-year-old patient has a prolonged febrile convulsion.

(a) What is the rectal dose of diazepam?
(i) 56 mg
(ii) 10 mg
(iii) 3 mg
(iv) 4.8 mg
(v) 5.6 mg

(b) What is the loading dose of phenytoin?
(i) 126 mg
(ii) 252 mg
(iii) 504 mg
(iv) 126 μg
(v) 252 μg

9.4 You are urgently called to A&E to see a six-week-old baby who is centrally cyanosed, but not in distress. The casualty officer has started facial oxygen and the saturations are 76%.

(a) What is the most likely diagnosis?

(b) What is your first action?

9.5 The following blood gas was obtained from a sick eight-year-old:

pH	7.15
Anion gap	40 mmol/L
K^+	5.7 mmol/L

What is the likely diagnosis?
(i) diabetic ketoacidosis
(ii) sepsis
(iii) proximal renal tubular acidosis
(iv) distal renal tubular acidosis
(v) aspirin overdose

9.6 A pre-term neonate is being ventilated for respiratory distress syndrome on the following setting:

Rate	60 b.p.m.
Inspiration	0.3 s
Pressure	24/4
O_2	40%

He is active and over the course of 15 min his oxygen requirement goes up.

His gas is:

pH	7.1
pCO_2	90 mmHg
pO_2	45 mmHg

(a) Give three possible explanations for this change.

(b) Give management instructions in appropriate order.

9.7 A neonate who has been ventilated for two days has a base deficit of 16. He has had a bolus of saline and you want to give him bicarbonate. His weight is 1.5 kg.

How much is a half correction of his acidosis?
   (i)   2 ml of 4.2%
   (ii)   4 ml of 4.2%
   (iii)   6 ml of 4.2%
   (iv)   8 ml of 4.2%
   (v)   10 ml of 4.2%

9.1 **(a)** (iii) (Age + 4) × 2 = 12 kg

(b) (iii) 0.1 ml/kg of 1 in 1000 = 1.2 ml
Comment: All emergency medicine follows national recognized guidelines – learn them.

9.2 **(a)** Check airway and breathing.

(b) First dose: 0.1 ml/kg of 1 in 10 000 = 1.8 ml
Subsequent dose: 1.8 ml of 1 in 1000.

9.3 **(a)** (v) 14 × 0.4 mg = 5.6 mg

(b) (ii) 14 × 18 mg = 252 mg, but only if not already on phenytoin
Comment: Writing the extra guide in **(b)** shows a greater understanding.

9.4 **(a)** Congenital heart disease.

(b) Stop the oxygen.
Comment: The child is blue but happy.

9.5 (i)
Comment: Acidosis with increased anion gap.

9.6 **(a)** Blocked/dislodged tube; pneumothorax; worsening disease.

(b) (1) Listen to air entry. (2) Cold light chest to exclude pneumothorax. (3) Reintubate as needed and then increase ventilation setting.
Comment: Think also sepsis and intraventricular haemorrhage. If there is coordination with the ventilator you may need to increase sedation.

9.7 (iv) 1.5 × ⅙ = 8 × 0.5 = 8 ml of 4.2% bicarbonate.

Helpful hints

BLOOD GASES

1. Always convert the gas into the units you are used to, using the factor 7.5.

   For example, mmHg = 7.5 × kPa.

2. Make sure the diagnosis fits the age of the patient.

   For example:

   Alkalosis in a six-week-old? Think pyloric stenosis.

   Alkalosis in a teenager? Think aspirin.

3. Decide whether the gas demonstrates a respiratory or a metabolic problem.

   If it is metabolic with normal anion gap it is either RTA or pyloric stenosis.

4. Neonatal causes:

Respiratory acidosis	Metabolic acidosis
RDS	Sepsis
Pneumothorax	Dehydrated
Blocked tube	Renal
Pneumonia	Metabolic
	Cardiac
	IVH

5. *NB*: Raised CO_2 with cyanosis is rarely cardiac.

9.8 A three-day-old with RDS is improving when you are asked to review the following arterial gas:

pH	7.29
pCO_2	70 mmHg
pO_2	80 mmHg
BE	−6 mmol/L

What would you like to do?

   (i)   increase the vent setting
  (ii)   saline bolus
 (iii)   repeat gas in one hour
 (iv)   bicarbonate bolus
  (v)   repeat gas

9.9 A six-hour-old 27-weeker is ventilated at a rate of 50 b.p.m. when you are asked to review the following gas:

pH	7.25
pCO_2	58 mmHg
pO_2	76 mmHg

The baby is in 60% oxygen and has intermittent uncoordinated respirations.

List three treatment options.

9.10 You are crash called to the emergency room where a four-year-old, who has fallen through the ice on a frozen pond, is in ventricular fibrillation.

(a) Give the appropriate defibrillation settings for three shocks:
   (i)   8   8   16
   (ii)   16   16   32
   (iii)   32   32   64
   (iv)   64   64   128
   (v)   128   128   256

(b) List three measures to warm him.

9.11 You are crash called to A&E to review a three-year-old boy who has been in a road traffic accident. You assess him using the paediatric Glasgow Coma Scale and demonstrate the following:

Eyes open to speech, verbal – cries to pain, flexing to pain

What total does this give?

   (i)   7
   (ii)   8
   (iii) 9
   (iv)   10
   (v)   11

9.12 The same boy now needs a fluid bolus. You want to give him normal saline.

Which volume is appropriate?

   (i)   260 ml
   (ii)   450 ml
   (iii) 900 ml
   (iv)   520 ml
   (v)   1000 ml

9.13 You are crash called to a six-year-old boy who is being bagged in A&E and needs intubating.

What size of tube would you like?

    (i)   6½
   (ii)   4
  (iii)   6
  (iv)   5½
   (v)   5

9.14 A four-year-old boy is intubated in A&E with meningococcal sepsis. You arrive with the transfer team. It is your hospital's policy to transfer children after nasal reintubation.

What length would you expect the ET to be?

    (i)   14
   (ii)   17
  (iii)   16
  (iv)   19
   (v)   20

9.15 A 10-year-old has been admitted to A&E with SVT on several occasions. You have tried vagal manoeuvres and one dose of adenosine without success.

What is your second dose of adenosine?

    (i)   2600 µg
   (ii)   2800 µg
  (iii)   26 mg
  (iv)   28 mg
   (v)   3000 µg

9.8 (v)
Comment: Raised CO_2 would need a positive base excess to have a pH of 7.29, so it must be wrong.

9.9 Increase the rate.

Increase the sedation.

Paralyse.
Comment: Try to decide the order you would use in practice.

9.10 **(a)** (iii)

$2 \times wt = 32$ J

$2 \times wt = 32$ J

$4 \times wt = 64$ J

(b) Remove wet clothing; warm blankets; warm i.v. fluids; peritoneal warming (or bladder/stomach); cardiac bypass.

NB: Do not use a space blanket – it keeps warm but does not warm.

9.11 (iii)
Comment: Easy to write questions on but not easy to remember.

9.12 (iv)
Comment: All fluid boluses are 20 ml/kg.

9.13 (iv)
Comment: With questions that are formula based, do the calculation and hopefully the answer will be there.

9.14 (i)

9.15 (ii)

Haematology

10

10.1 Further investigation of a three-year-old with suspected platelet disease has the following results:

On film, platelets appear normal

Normal aggregation to ADP and collagen

But abnormal aggregation to ristocetin

What is the likely diagnosis?

    (i)   Bernard–Soulier disease
    (ii)   ITP
   (iii) haemophilia
   (iv) von Willebrand's disease
    (v)   DIC

10.2 A four-month-old is thought to be pale when seen by a GP.

A full blood count is taken:

Hb	4.6 g/dl
WCC	11.2×10^9/L
Platelets	225×10^9/L
Reticulocytes	0.5%

(a) Suggest a possible diagnosis:
    (i) iron deficiency
    (ii) leukaemia
    (iii) malaria
    (iv) Blackfan–Diamond syndrome
    (v) lead poisoning

(b) How would you confirm it?

10.3 A four-year-old being investigated for anaemia had the following electrophoresis results:

HbA	85%
HbA_2	5%
HbF	3%

What is the reason for his anaemia?

    (i) β-thalassaemia trait
    (ii) α-thalassaemia trait
    (iii) iron deficiency
    (iv) normal
    (v) β-thalassaemia major

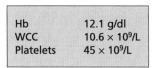

10.4 A six-year-old boy suffering from recurrent infections with associated eczema has his FBC checked:

Hb	12.1 g/dl
WCC	10.6 × 10⁹/L
Platelets	45 × 10⁹/L

(a) What is the likely diagnosis?
  (i) histiocytosis
  (ii) SCID
  (iii) Wiskott–Aldrich syndrome
  (iv) recovering ITP with eczema
  (v) poor sample

(b) What are the immunoglobulin levels (IgA, IgE, IgM)?

10.5 An Asian child is suspected of having α-thalassaemia. FBC shows he has a mean cell haemoglobin (MCH) of 30 pg.

Does he need further investigation?

10.6 You are asked to see a two-year-old girl who complains of back pain and has a history of frequent illness. Her mother feels she has been pale for about six months.

FBC:

Hb	5.7 g/dl
WCC	7.3 × 10⁹/L
Platelets	352 × 10⁹/L
MCV	78 fl
Blood film	normal

(a) What is your primary concern?
  (i) Blackfan–Diamond syndrome
  (ii) SCID
  (iii) malignancy
  (iv) infection
  (v) iron deficiency anaemia

(b) List two further investigations you would make.

10.7 You are asked to see a child with a rash. Your clinical diagnosis is urticarial but because of marked bruising you ask for an FBC:

Hb	9.3 g/dl
WCC	10.4 × 10⁹/L
Platelets	232 × 10⁹/L
MCH	22.4 pg
MCV	69.6 fl
Zinc protoporphyrin	63 µmol ZPP/mol haem
HbA₂	3.9 (2.1–3.4%)
HbF	2.6 (<0.8%)

(a) What is the diagnosis?
- (i) α-thalassaemia
- (ii) β-thalassaemia
- (iii) iron deficiency anaemia
- (iv) β-thalassaemia with iron deficiency
- (v) α-thalassaemia with iron deficiency

(b) Can this present as neonatal jaundice?

10.8 You review a three-year-old with lower back pain who has poor appetite and drinks 4–5 pints of milk a day. She is thriving.

The results of an FBC:

Hb	10.1 g/L
WCC	4.4 × 10⁹/L
Platelets	227 × 10⁹/L
MCV	68.5 fl

(a) What is the likely diagnosis?
- (i) iron deficiency
- (ii) β-thalassaemia
- (iii) Blackfan–Diamond syndrome
- (iv) sepsis
- (v) leukaemia

(b) What confirmatory blood test is there?

10.9 You are reviewing a four-year-old with bruises. There is a history of a pyrexial illness with red cheeks:

Hb	12.6 g/dL
WCC	2.5×10^9/L
Platelets	10×10^9/L

(a) What illness has she had?
  (i) 1st disease of childhood
  (ii) 6th disease of childhood
  (iii) 2nd disease of childhood
  (iv) 4th disease of childhood
  (v) 5th disease of childhood

(b) What is the causative agent?
  (i) parvovirus B 19
  (ii) adenovirus
  (iii) Herpesvirus type VI
  (iv) Herpesvirus type I
  (v) RSV

10.10 You are asked to see a 10-year-old child in out-patients whose father is Chinese. He has presented with non-specific abdominal pain:

Hb	11.8 g/dl
MCV	70.6 fl
MCH	22.1 pg
HbA$_2$	2.8 (normal 2.1–3.4%)
HbF	0.5 (<0.8%)
Zinc protoporphyrin	43 (normal 0–80) μmol ZPP/mol haem
Film	microcytosis, hypochromia

(a) What is the likely diagnosis?

    (i)   G6PD deficiency

    (ii) β-thalassaemia

    (iii) sickle cell

    (iv) α-thalassaemia

    (v) iron deficiency

(b) Is it causing her abdominal pain?

(c) What neonatal problems may it cause?

10.11 You are asked to see a jaundiced baby on day 1:

Bilirubin	110 μmol/L
Baby's blood group	O Rh-positive
Mother's blood group	O Rh-negative

Mother tells you that she has had a splenectomy.

(a) Give two possible diagnoses.

(b) Give two differentiating tests.

10.12 You are reviewing a thriving two-year-old in clinic with a 2 cm spleen and a family history of spherocytosis.

FBC results:

Hb	9.0 g/dl
WCC	10.4 × 10⁹/L
MCV	29 fl
Platelets	422 × 10⁹/L
Zinc protoporphyrin	87 (0–80) μmol ZPP/mol haem
Reticulocytes	10.2%

(a) Name one medication this child should be given:
  (i)   iron
  (ii) folic acid
  (iii) multi-vitamins
  (iv) penicillin
  (v)   B$_{12}$

(b) If this child needs a splenectomy give two management requirements.

10.13 A two-year-old has been in for six days with a pyrexia, cough and a fine macular rash which seems to appear with the evening rise in temperature. Palpable spleen 2 cm:

Hb	8.1 g/dl
WCC	17.4 × 10⁹/L
MCV	70.6 fl
Platelets	606 × 10⁹/L
ESR	120 mm/h

(a) What is the most likely diagnosis?
  (i)   leukaemia
  (ii) malaria
  (iii) systemic juvenile arthritis
  (iv) tuberculosis
  (v)   Kawasaki's syndrome

(b) What would be your initial treatment?

10.14 A 2½-year-old with Still's disease is not well controlled so is admitted for a bone marrow biopsy.

    (a) Why has he had a bone marrow biopsy?

    (b) How would you monitor the Still's disease?

10.15 You are asked to take over the care of a term neonate under double lights for a high bilirubin. Its blood group is AB negative and the DCT is positive. The mother is also AB negative.

Which of the following blood groups can the father not be?

    (i)   A negative
   (ii)   O negative
  (iii)   A positive
  (iv)   AB positive
   (v)   B negative

10.16 You are reviewing a three-day-old baby on the postnatal wards. The mother wants to know whether the baby has passive immunization from her. For which of the following, if the mother has had, will the child not have passive immunization?

    (i)   chickenpox
   (ii)   herpes
  (iii)   whooping cough
  (iv)   rubella
   (v)   HIV

10.17 A six-year-old boy with a family history of bruising comes to see you. You suspect he has von Willebrand's disease and so order the following tests.

Which two would most help to confirm the diagnosis?

    (i)   platelet count
   (ii)   bleeding time
  (iii)   PT
  (iv)   APPT
   (v)   factor VIII levels
  (vi)   factor IX levels
 (vii)   ristocetin-induced platelet aggregation

10.18 A four-day-old neonate goes off with what is believed to be sepsis. One of the nurses is checking the baby's blood glucose and comments that the heel is still bleeding 10 minutes later:

	Bleeding time	PT	APTT	TT	Fibrinogen
(i)	→→	→	→	↓	
(ii)	↑	↑	↑	↑	↓
(iii)	↑	→	↑	→	→
(iv)	→	→↑	→	→	
(v)	→	↑	→↑	↑	→

(a) Which of the above would suggest the baby has DIC?

(b) Which of the above would suggest haemophilia?

10.19 You are asked to see a 10-day-old girl whose cord fell off on day 6 but the cord has been oozing ever since. You order the following tests:

Platelets – normal

PT – normal

APPT – normal

Bleeding time – normal

Which of the following may be deficient?

    (i)   plasminogen
    (ii)   factor VII
    (iii)   vitamin K
    (iv)   factor XIII
    (v)   factor IX

10.20 A nine-year-old boy presents with bruises. He is otherwise well. You have excluded ITP and leukaemia. You suspect he has haemophilia. Which of the following levels of factor VIII would be consistent with moderate levels?

    (i)   0–1%
    (ii)   1–5%
    (iii)   5–10%
    (iv)   10–20%
    (v)   20–50%

10.21 You are looking after a newborn baby on the neonatal unit. He has suspected pneumonia and you have ordered an FBC. What is the normal range for his mean cell volume?

    (i)   80–90
   (ii)   90–100
  (iii)   100–110
  (iv)   110–120
   (v)   120–130

10.1 **(a)** (iv)
Comment: Normal-size platelets; if large then consider Bernard–Soulier disease.

10.2 **(a)** (iv)

(b) Bone marrow biopsy.
Comment: Best fit to age; may also mention hypoplasia of the thumb.

10.3 (i)
Comment: The presence of HbF tells you it is β and the presence of HbA tells you it is trait.

10.4 **(a)** (iii)

(b) IgA ↑, IgE ↑, IgM ↓.
Comment: There is a group of syndromes with altered immunoglobulin levels but there is no logic to them so they have to be learnt.

10.5 No.
Comment: You only need to investigate if it is less than 27 pg.

10.6 **(a)** (iii)

(b) MRI scan of spine; bone marrow biopsy.
Comment: It is very unusual for a child to complain of back pain. It may also be infection, but in view of the low haemoglobin the prime concern is malignancy.

10.7 **(a)** (ii)

(b) No.
Comment: Increased HbA_2 + HbF β chains are not present at birth so do not cause neonatal problems.

10.8 **(a)** (i)

(b) Zinc protoporphyrin levels or ferritin levels.
Comment: Milk allows a baby to thrive but is a very poor source of iron.

10.9 **(a)** (v) (also known as slapped cheek syndrome or erythema infectiosum)

(b) (i)

10.10 **(a)** (iv)

(b) No.

(c) Neonatal hydrops; intrauterine death.
Comment: Low normal haemoglobin with a very low mean cell haemoglobin is usually either thalassaemia or iron deficiency.

10.11 **(a)** Rhesus incompatibility; spherocytosis.

(b) Direct Coombs test; blood film; red cell fragility test.
Comment: In **(a)** the order is probably not relevant as both are likely. In **(b)** two tests are needed that differentiate between your diagnosis in **(a)**.

10.12 **(a)** (ii) (fewer marks for iron)

(b) Pneumococcal/meningococcal/haemophilus B vaccination – encapsulated organisms; prophylactic penicillin.
Comment: The reticulocyte count is much higher than the zinc protoporphyrin level. In **(b)**, do not put down two vaccinations.

10.13 **(a)** (iii)

(b) NSAIDs.
Comment: Evening rise of temperature is the clue here.

10.14 **(a)** To exclude leukaemia before starting oral steroids.

(b) ESR; platelets; clinically.
Comment: All children who are going on to steroids need a biopsy – that includes those with idiopathic thrombocytopenia purpura (ITP).

10.15 (ii)
Comment: This is the sort of question that just needs to be written down.

10.16 (iii)
Comment: This can be worked out, e.g. which illness would cause most problems for a month-old baby?

10.17 (ii, vii)
Comment: Cross off the answers you know are wrong.

10.18 **(a)** (ii)

(b) (iv)
Comment: Sorry – no easy way to do this. Just work your way through each line.

10.19 (iv)

10.20 (ii)

10.21 (iv)
Comment: It is worth knowing which variables change with age, as then one can assume the rest don't.

Gastro-enterology

QUESTIONS

11.1 You are reviewing a two-year-old with a family history of coeliac disease, who is not thriving:

Total protein	50 g/L
IgA	<0.2 g/L
Anti-endomysial antibodies	not detected

Please comment.

11.2 A four-week-old is referred because of mild jaundice. She is breast-fed and feeding well:

Bilirubin total	110 µmol/L
Indirect	20 µmol/L

What is the most likely diagnosis?

11.3 You are requested to do the following investigation on a three-year-old who is chesty:

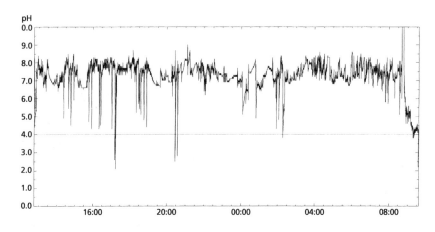

(a) What is the investigation?

(b) Have you found the reason for his chestiness?

11.4 The tracing below was taken from a child who has been having frequent absences. These were thought to have been caused by reflux:

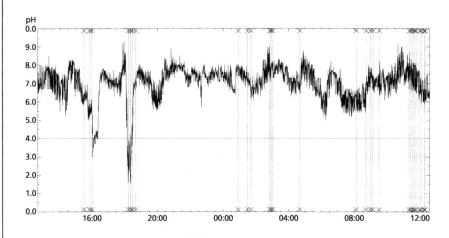

(a) Are there any indications of reflux?

(b) Is reflux the cause of these episodes?

11.5 The child below has cerebral palsy. He is to have a percutaneous endoscopic gastrostomy (PEG):

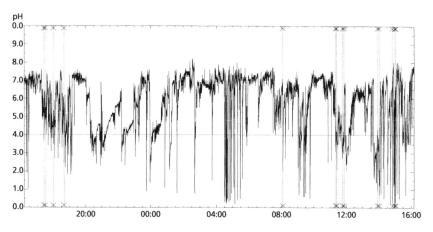

(a) Is he having the right operation?

(b) Justify your answer.

11.6 You are reviewing a six-month-old baby with constipation. There is some improvement with lactulose and senna. Reviewing his notes he was initially breast-fed and first opened his bowels on day 6. What would you do next?

    (i)   continue
    (ii)   rule out coeliac disease
    (iii) rule out Hirschsprung's disease
    (iv) rule out hypothyroidism
    (v)   rule out CF.

11.7 A four-year-old with an acute abdomen has the following findings:
Abdomen: tender on the right, bowel sounds present.
FBC:

Hb	15 g/dl
WCC	20×10^9/L (90% neutrophils)
Platelets	400×10^9/L
Amylase	650 IU/L
Ultrasound	free fluid – 2.5 cm mass behind the bladder

(a) What is the diagnosis?

(b) Give two possible aetiologies.

(c) Give one complication.

11.8 A 14-year-old girl presents with anorexia and weight loss. She has some painful lesions on her shins. The rest of the examination is unremarkable. You suspect erythema nodosum.

Which of the following causes would be top of your list?

(i)   the pill
(ii) mycoplasma
(iii) Crohn's disease
(iv) sarcoid
(v)   strep throat

11.9 A 10-year-old girl with good diabetic control starts to fail to thrive. You have checked her TFTs; they are normal.

Which of the following would most likely give an explanation?

(i)   Hb A1C
(ii) LH/FSH
(iii) Anti-endomysial antibodies
(iv) GH
(v)   CF screen

11.10 You have been reviewing an eight-year-old girl with abdominal pain and intermittent diarrhoea. There is no history of weight loss and she looks well. You have done a few baseline investigations which are all normal. You believe she has irritable bowel syndrome.

What type of diarrhoea is this?

(i)   secretory
(ii) osmotic
(iii) decreased surface area
(iv) increased motility
(v)   mucosa invasion

11.11 You are called to see a six-hour-old baby because he choked and vomited his first feed. He has lots of secretions. You suspect an oesophageal atresia. X-ray with repogal tube confirms the diagnosis. There is no air in the stomach. Which of the following could it be (pick two)?

(i)   type A
(ii) type B
(iii) type C
(iv) type D
(v)   type E

11.12 You see a six-week-old baby because the health visitor is worried. He is fully breast-fed and beginning to smile. He has no diarrhoea but possets a lot and has only put on 90 g in the last week. You suspect he has significant reflux and start him on Gaviscon.

If you are successful, what would be an appropriate weight gain each week?
- (i) 120 g
- (ii) 150 g
- (iii) 180 g
- (iv) 210 g
- (v) 240 g

11.13 Matthew is admitted to the acute ward with a seven-day history of bloody diarrhoea and vomiting. He is apyrexial but has generalized tenderness. Initial results are:

Hb	13.2
WCC	12.9
Na	135
K	3.5
HCO$_3$	18
Stool culture	negative

(a) What is the most likely diagnosis?
- (i) salmonella
- (ii) amoebic dysentery
- (iii) coeliac disease
- (iv) Crohn's disease
- (v) ulcerative colitis

(b) What is the investigation to confirm?
- (i) repeat stool cultures
- (ii) small bowel meal
- (iii) jejunal biopsy
- (iv) barium enema
- (v) colonoscopy and biopsy

(c) What is the treatment of choice?
- (i) metronidazole
- (ii) remove gluten
- (iii) i.v. steroids
- (iv) oral steroids
- (v) supportive

11.1 Anti-endomysial is IgA, so as the IgA levels are very low it is not a useful test. The child needs a jejunal biopsy.

11.2 Biliary atresia.
Comment: Do not be fooled when you are given results that you are not used to, for example indirect bilirubin.

11.3 (a) 24 h oesophageal pH.

(b) No.
Comment: Now you have seen a 24 h reading then the pH readings will be easy.

11.4 (a) Minimal evidence, as only two episodes are below pH 4.0.

(b) No: the lines are episodes of absence and they are not related to reflux.

11.5 (a) No.

(b) The 24 h pH recording has demonstrated numerous episodes of reflux. It is not possible to perform an anti-reflux procedure such as Nissan's with an endoscope. Reflux should normally be less than 10% of the total times.

11.6 (iii) Take a rectal biopsy to rule out Hirschsprung's.

11.7 (a) Pancreatitis.

(b) Mumps; cystic fibrosis; trauma.

(c) Pseudocyst.

Comment: This question is easy if you put next to each answer 'high', 'low' or 'normal'.

11.8 (iii)
Comment: Erythema nodosum with anorexia and weight loss. Make sure answer fits with all three.

11.9 (iii)

Comment: Coeliac disease is associated with Down's syndrome.

11.10 (iv) Try to think of examples of the others.

Comment: Examples – osmotic, laxative abuse, coeliac disease, decreased surface area, short gut.

11.11 (i, iii)

11.12 (iv)

11.13 **(a)** (v)

 (b) (v)

 (c) (iii)

Comment: Another good example of crossing out answers, e.g. culture negative so unlikely to be salmonella.

Syndromes

12

12.1 A three-week-old baby presents with vomiting and diarrhoea. An observant SHO notices lens clouding.

    (a) What is the most likely diagnosis?
       (i)   rubella
      (ii) galactosaemia
     (iii) tyrosinaemia
     (iv) hypothyroidism
      (v) renal tubular acidosis

    (b) Name a confirmatory test.

12.2 A three-year-old child with learning difficulties is referred to you by the ophthalmologist.

    (a) What is the most likely diagnosis?
       (i)   Marfan's syndrome
      (ii) galactosaemia
     (iii) Tay–Sachs disease
     (iv) homocystinuria
      (v) cerebral palsy

    (b) Name a confirmatory test on the urine.

12.3 A 10-year-old is referred to you for intermittent mild jaundice. His urine and stools are normal.

  (a) What is the most likely diagnosis?
- (i) hepatitis B
- (ii) Gilbert's syndrome
- (iii) Dubin–Johnson syndrome
- (iv) Rotor's syndrome
- (v) hepatitis A

  (b) What is the mode of inheritance?
- (i) sporadic
- (ii) X-linked dominant
- (iii) X-linked recessive
- (iv) autosomal dominant
- (v) autosomal recessive

12.4 A seven-year-old girl is referred with tiredness and symmetrical proximal muscle weakness. There is some tenderness.

  (a) Give two other features you would look for.

  (b) What is the mainstay of treatment?
- (i) paracetamol
- (ii) splinting
- (iii) steroids
- (iv) interferon
- (v) ibuprofen

12.5 You are asked to see a three-year-old boy who has pubic hair and an enlarged penis. His electrolytes, however, are normal.

What is the most likely diagnosis?

- (i) congenital adrenal hyperplasia
- (ii) congenital adrenal hypoplasia
- (iii) central precocious puberty
- (iv) adrenal tumour
- (v) normal

12.1 **(a)** (ii)

(b) Galactose-1-phosphate uridyl transferase (Gal-I-PUT) blood test.
Comment: Give the full test names.

12.2 **(a)** (iv)

(b) Homocystine levels.
Comment: Other syndromes have eye changes, but the diagnosis needs to be made on a urine sample.

12.3 **(a)** (ii)

(b) (v)

12.4 **(a)** Facial purple heliotrope rash; oedema in hands or feet; subcutaneous nodules.

(b) (iii)
Comment: The child has dermatomyositis.

12.5 (i)
Comment: Use all the information in the question. Adrenal pubertal growth does not affect the testes or ovaries as they are controlled by LH/FSH.

Helpful hints

SYNDROMES

1. The syndromes that you remember are the ones that you have seen.

2. To facilitate this there are two options:

    (a) Go to your local special schools even before the clinical part of this examination.

    (b) After answering any question on syndromes take notes, then look in the syndrome book.

3. **2(a)** is the best option as most syndromes that you will be asked about rarely come in as patients.

4. These questions are quite common in the slide section and hint no. **2** helps because features run true. It is not wasted time.

12.6 A seven-year-old with acne is referred to you. You notice that she is obese.

    (a) What is the most likely diagnosis?
       (i)   precocious puberty
      (ii) Addison's disease
     (iii) Conn's syndrome
     (iv) Cushing's syndrome
      (v) congenital adrenal hyperplasia

    (b) Give two other clinical features.

12.7 A 13-year-old girl is referred to you through the school nurse because she looks tired although she says she doesn't feel it.

    (a) What is a possible diagnosis?
       (i)   chronic fatigue syndrome
      (ii) drug abuse
     (iii) myasthenia gravis
     (iv) normal
      (v) myotonia

    (b) Give two treatment options.

12.8 You are referred an eight-year-old boy who has hypermobile joints. There is a history of numerous abscesses.

(a) What is the most likely diagnosis?
- (i) Job's syndrome
- (ii) Ehlers–Danlos syndrome
- (iii) Marfan's syndrome
- (iv) Homocystinuria
- (v) SCID

(b) Name one possible treatment.
- (i) regular immunoglobulins
- (ii) cimetidine
- (iii) routine antibiotics
- (iv) antiseptic soap
- (v) leave alone

12.9 You are reviewing a child with obesity in the follow-up clinic. Reading his notes you see that a plastic surgeon has seen him for polydactyly. He has also been diagnosed as having visual problems.

(a) What is the underlying diagnosis?

(b) Explain his visual problems.
- (i) retinitis pigmentosa
- (ii) cherry red spot
- (iii) corneal clouding
- (iv) cataract
- (v) papilloedema

12.10 You are asked to see an 18-month-old who was developing normally until seven months of age. Autism has been suggested but the child's condition is getting worse. There are hyperventilation episodes and head growth has slowed.

(a) What is the diagnosis?
- (i) Lesch–Nyhan syndrome
- (ii) rubella
- (iii) Asperger's syndrome
- (iv) familial microcephaly
- (v) Rett's syndrome

(b) What sex is the child?

12.11 A six-week-old baby is coming for routine follow-up. She was growth retarded and on the neonatal screen failed her hearing test. She continues to fail to thrive and her mother is worried because she does not appear to look at her. You suspect she has congenital rubella.

Which of the following eye changes would you not expect?

- (i) chorioretinitis
- (ii) retinitis pigmentosa
- (iii) cataracts
- (iv) glaucoma
- (v) corneal clouding

12.12 You are reviewing a six-hour-old baby with growth retardation and petechiae. Examination of the eyes reveals glaucoma.

Which of the following is most likely?

- (i) toxoplasmosis
- (ii) rubella
- (iii) CMV
- (iv) herpes
- (v) enterovirus

12.13 You are reviewing a four-year-old boy for assessment. He has significant pubic hair growth and penile enlargement although his testes are small. On plotting him on the centile charts he is on the 97th centile. You diagnose pseudo-precocious puberty.

Which of the following tests will be of least use?

- (i) urinary steroids
- (ii) bone age
- (iii) abdominal ultrasound
- (iv) serum 17-hydroxyprogesterone levels
- (v) MRI head

12.14 You are called to the high-dependency unit, where a six-day-old has just arrived. She is semi-conscious and has fitted. There is also a history of some vomiting. The blood glucose is low and you suspect the baby has maple syrup urine disease.

Which of the following tests is used to confirm the diagnosis?

    (i)   urinary and blood amino acids
    (ii)   urinary organic acids
   (iii)   skin fibroblasts
   (iv)   urinary amino acids and organic acids
    (v)   urinary ketoacidosis

12.15 A two-week-old is continuing to cause concern on the neonatal unit. He is drowsy and difficult to feed. He is also significantly hypotonic. The nurses feel he is fitting. Having excluded many metabolic problems your consultant speaks to the regional centre. They suggest you rule out non-ketotic hyperglycinaemia. What paired sample do you need to send?

    (i)   blood and urine
    (ii)   CSF and urine
   (iii)   CSF and blood
   (iv)   blood and stools
    (v)   stools and urine

12.16 Bethany was admitted to SCBU because of prolonged resuscitation. She had been intubated for 15 minutes. She settled very quickly on SCBU and, although she looked slightly dysmorphic, her mother said she looked like her other children. She was due to be seen in out-patients at 6/52 and because of the neonatal period had two hearing tests, which she had failed. At three weeks she was admitted with a cold and she had lost 300 g. On examination she had an antimongoloid slant and high palate and small lower jaw. There was no defect with the eyes and the ears were slightly small and primitive. The geneticist came to look and said she looks classical.

(a) Which syndrome is this?
  (i) Alagille's
  (ii) Down's
  (iii) Pierre Robin's
  (iv) Williams'
  (v) Stickler's

(b) What would you expect her IQ to be?
  (i) normal
  (ii) low normal
  (iii) mild mental retardation
  (iv) moderate mental retardation
  (v) severe mental retardation

12.17 Mark is nine and referred by his GP for polyuria and polydipsia. He has also been losing weight for the last five months. He drinks mostly in the evening but also at night. His blood results are as follows:

Hb	12.9
WCC	7.0
Platelets	366
Glu	6.3
Na	134
K	4.6
U	3.2
Creatinine	56

(a) What is the likely diagnosis?
  (i)   psychogenic polydipsia
  (ii) diabetes insipidus
  (iii) diabetes mellitus
  (iv) anorexia
  (v)   UTI

(b) What investigation would you do?
  (i)   morning urine
  (ii) water deprivation test
  (iii) trial of DDAVP
  (iv) urine for MC & S
  (v)   none

12.6 **(a)** (iv)

(b) Stretch marks; hirsutism.
Comment: Increased BP would not be a clinical feature.

12.7 **(a)** (iii)

(b) Neostigmine; thymectomy.
Comment: Thymectomy fits with female sex.

12.8 **(a)** (i)

(b) (ii)
Comment: It is also known as hyper-IgE syndrome.

12.9 **(a)** Laurence–Moon–Biedl.

(b) (i)

12.10 **(a)** (v)

(b) Female.
Comment: When asked what sex a child is, do not assume the child is male!

12.11 (ii)
Comment: Always read questions carefully as the word `not' is the crucial one.

12.12 (ii)
Comment: If you read any of the answers and know their typical finding then cross them out.

12.13 (v)
Comment: Pseudo-precocious puberty is non-central in origin.

12.14 (iii)
Comment: Clue – the word 'confirm'.

12.15 (iii)

12.16 (a) (iv)

(b) (i)
Comment: Some syndromes are obvious at birth but most are not and then some are retrospectively obvious, e.g. Prader–Willi and neonatal hypotonia.

12.17 (a) (i)

(b) (i)
Comment: Normal electrolytes are unlikely to have pathology.

Neonates

13.1 A 32-week-old neonate has the following vent settings: 40 b.p.m., 0.3 s, 18/4, 50%, when you are doing the following gas:

pH	7.24
pCO$_2$	6.0
PO$_2$	5.7
HCO$_3$	20
BE	−3.0

What alteration would you like to do?

(i)   increase rate
(ii)   increase inspiratory time
(iii)   increase pressure
(iv)   saline bolus
(v)   repeat in 1 hour

13.2 A 26-week-old neonate on the ventilator is on 60 b.p.m., 0.34 s, 18/4, when you do the following gas:

pH	7.23
pCO_2	4.1
pO_2	7.9
HCO_3	17
BE	−8

What will you do?

(i)   treat the base deficit
(ii) repeat the gas
(iii) increase the vent and treat the base deficit
(iv) increase the vent
(v)   decrease the vent and treat the base deficit

13.3 A term neonate is born weighing 1.8 kg. On examination there are no murmurs and ears are not low set. There is some overlapping of fingers and he is hungry.

What test is top of the list?

(i)   gas
(ii) TORCH screen
(iii) Screen for Down's
(iv) eye examination
(v)   screen for Edwards' syndrome

13.4 A mother is asking you about the Guthrie test.

Which of the following will not be covered?

(i)   thyroid dyshormonogenesis
(ii) absent thyroid
(iii) central hypothyroidism
(iv) cystic fibrosis
(v)   phenylketonuria

13.5 You are checking the results of a neonate.

Which of the following has a different normal range from adults?

(i)   sodium
(ii) potassium
(iii) phosphate
(iv) urea
(v)   glucose

13.6 You are discussing vitamins with the dietitian and you are particularly interested in antioxidants.

Which of the following is an antioxidant?

(i)   vitamin K
(ii) vitamin D
(iii) vitamin B_6
(iv) vitamin B_{12}
(v)   vitamin E

13.7 You are doing a metabolic screen on the neonatal unit.

Which of the following tests has to be sent on ice?

(i)   lactate
(ii) venous gas
(iii) ammonia
(iv) Gal-I-PUT
(v)   amino acid screen

13.8 You are speaking to parents-to-be of a potential 23-weeker who want to know the prognosis. The survival rate is:

(i)   1%
(ii) 5%
(iii) 10%
(iv) 25%
(v)   45%

13.9 You are reviewing the vitamin K policy for the newborn.

Which of the following is right when comparing the different types?

    (i)   vitamin K i.m. is best
    (ii) vitamin K oral is best
    (iii) vitamin K i.v. is best
    (iv) vitamin K i.m. or i.v. is best
    (v) all are equally as good

13.10 You are asked to give a 2 kg baby sodium supplements for low sodium. The registrar asks for 4 mmol/kg/day.

Which is the right dose of 30%?

    (i)   0.4 ml q.d.s.
    (ii) 0.2 ml q.d.s.
    (iii) 0.5 ml q.d.s.
    (iv) 0.2 ml b.d.
    (v) 0.5 ml b.d.

13.11 You are reviewing a baby on day 3 with what you believe is physiological jaundice.

Which of the following is relevant to pathological jaundice only?

    (i)   increase destruction
    (ii) decreased life span
    (iii) altered binding
    (iv) decreased albumin
    (v) increased enterohepatic shunting

13.12 The energy requirements of a premature baby are being looked at as a part of the neonatal ward round. The infant needs approximately 120 kcal/kg/day.

How many calories does a premature infant expend at rest?

    (i)   5
    (ii) 10
    (iii) 20
    (iv) 50
    (v) 100

13.13 You are discussing passive immunization by IgG transfer from the mother to a woman in early labour.

At what gestation does efficient transport begin?

    (i)   24 weeks
   (ii)   28 weeks
  (iii)   30 weeks
  (iv)   32 weeks
   (v)   34 weeks

13.14 You are reviewing the serology of a mother who is known to be hepatitis B positive.

Which of the following shows the highest infection risk?

    (i)   HBs Ag
   (ii)   HBe Ag
  (iii)   Anti-HBe
  (iv)   Anti-HBs
   (v)   HBs Ag and HBe Ag

13.1 (ii)
Comment: This is the inspiratory time of a 24-weeker.

13.2 (v)
Comment: CO_2 less than 5 can increase the risk of chronic lung disease, so although the gas is acidotic it must be acted on.

13.3 (v)
Comment: You cannot ignore the overlapping fingers although nothing else is seen.

13.4 (iii)
Comment: This type is very rare but is covered by screening in America.

13.5 (iii)
Comment: This tends to be higher in neonates.

13.6 (v)

13.7 (i)

13.8 (iii)
Comment: This is epicure data and if there is one neonatal paper to read this is it.

13.9 (i)
Comment: It acts as a depot.

13.10 (i)
Comment: 30% NaC1 is 5 mmol/ml and note it is a 2 kg baby.

13.11 (i)
Comment: (ii) (iv) (v) are all physiological and (iii) can be either pathological or physiological.

13.12 (iv)
Comment: Almost half their energy.

13.13 (iii)
Comment: They do start crossing at 8 weeks.

13.14 (ii)

Miscellaneous

14

14.1 A 12-year-old boy presents to you with a painful left leg. There is some restriction of movement.

    (a) What is the most likely diagnosis?
        (i) irritable hip
        (ii) pathological fracture
        (iii) septic arthritis
        (iv) Perthes' disease
        (v) Slipped femoral epiphysis

    (b) What is the investigation of choice?

14.2 A three-year-old presents with a limp and pain that wakes her at night. The hip X-ray is normal and so are the FBC and ESR.

    What is the next investigation?

14.3

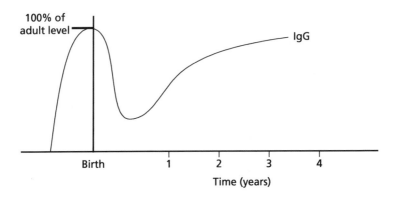

Explain the Ig levels in the graph.

14.4 A child can lift his leg against gravity but not if there is added resistance.

What muscle strength is this?

    (i)   1/5
    (ii) 2/5
    (iii) 3/5
    (iv) 4/5
    (v) 5/5

14.5 A GP has asked you to see a toddler with a painless swelling above his right eye.

(a) Suggest a diagnosis.

    (i)   sebaceous cyst
    (ii) dermoid
    (iii) infected sweat gland
    (iv) entropia
    (v) lipoma

(b) Name one other site.

14.6 A baby is born with a swelling of the left side of the scrotum. Over the next 24 h it goes blue/black.

    (a) What is the diagnosis?
        (i)   congenital torsion
        (ii) hydrocele
        (iii) obstructed hernia
        (iv) non-obstructed hernia
        (v) haemangioma

    (b) What is the prognosis?

    (c) Does the child need an operation?

14.7 Two children have their visual fields tested.

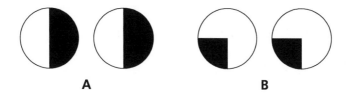

         A   **B**

    (a) Where is the lesion in child A?
        (i)   optic chiasm
        (ii) left optic tract
        (iii) right optic tract
        (iv) left optic nerve
        (v) right optic nerve

    (b) Where is the lesion in child B?
        (i)   optic chiasm
        (ii) right temporal lobe radiation
        (iii) left temporal lobe radiation
        (iv) right parietal lobe radiation
        (v) left parietal lobe radiation

14.8 You are asked to review the following cell count from a lumbar puncture undertaken on a 12-year-old boy:

RBC	214 000 × 10⁶/L
WBC	396 × 10⁶/L

Is it significant?

14.9 A nine-year-old girl initially presents with some facial weakness. The following lumbar puncture result is available:

WCC	< 5 × 10⁶/L
Protein	2.2 g/L
Glucose	3.6 mmol/L

   (a) What is the diagnosis?
      (i) viral meningitis
      (ii) Bell's palsy
      (iii) Guillain–Barré syndrome
      (iv) multiple sclerosis
      (v) partially treated meningitis

   (b) What monitoring is most important?

14.10 A 15-month-old is admitted; she is refusing to walk and has prominence of the spine in the thoraco-lumbar area. She is apyrexial and not distressed.

FBC:

Hb	11.4 g/dL
WCC	11.5 × 10⁹/L
Platelets	415 × 10⁹/L
CRP	12 mg/L
Plain X-ray of spine erosion	L1–L2

What are the main differential diagnoses?

14.11 You are taking over the care of a term infant with meconium aspiration. It is 12 hours old and in 90% oxygen. The vent is set at 50 b.p.m. with pressures of 30/4 mean 14.

An arterial gas has an O_2 of 6 kPa. What is the oxygen index?

    (i)   14
    (ii)   28
    (iii)   32
    (iv)   20
    (v)   49

14.12 You are writing new guidelines for the management of hypoglycaemia on the postnatal wards.

Which of the following is the cut-off for hypoglycaemia?

    (i)   2
    (ii)   2.5
    (iii)   2.7
    (iv)   3.0
    (v)   1.0

14.13 You are doing a septic screen on a term neonate for PROM. This includes an LP.

Up to what number of white cells is acceptable?

    (i)   <10
    (ii)   <20
    (iii)   <30
    (iv)   <40
    (v)   <50

14.14 You are discussing the prognosis with a mother and father on the postnatal wards. The baby had been diagnosed as having Down's syndrome two days before.

    (a) Which of the following complications is most frequent?
        (i)   gastrointestinal abnormalities
        (ii)   congenital heart disease
        (iii) hypothyroidism
        (iv) leukaemia
        (v)   hearing loss

    (b) At what age are they most likely to get leukaemia?
        (i)   less than 6 months
        (ii)   2–3 years
        (iii) 5–10 years
        (iv) teenagers
        (v)   as adults

14.15 You are seeing a couple who have a family history of haemophilia. They have come for antenatal counselling.

    (a) Which of the following family trees fits with the condition?

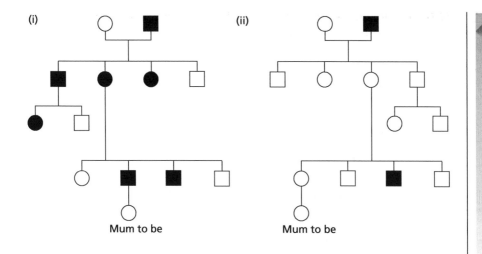

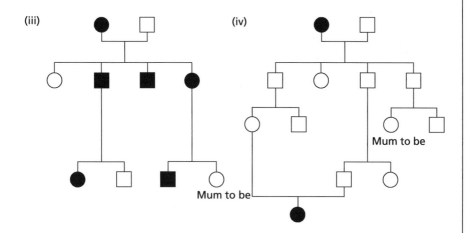

(b) What is the chance of her male offspring having the condition?
  (i)   none
  (ii)   1/2
  (iii)   1/4
  (iv)   1/8
  (v)   1/16

14.16 A three-year-old presents to you having had a cold a couple of weeks before. He was noted at school to have bruises on knees and arms. The teacher was worried that there are some petechiae but there is no hepatosplenomegaly.

    (a) Which of the following is most likely?
        (i)   non-accidental injury
        (ii) idiopathic thrombocytopenia purpura
        (iii) leukaemia
        (iv) Henoch–Schönlein purpura
        (v) childhood injuries

    (b) Which is the most appropriate treatment?
        (i)   immunoglobulins
        (ii) case conference
        (iii) steroids
        (iv) no treatment
        (v) antibiotics

14.17 A 10-year-old girl comes in with diarrhoea and abdominal pain. Initial examination shows she is pyrexial with a small node in her neck and a soft abdomen. Her BP is 128/70. Initial tests show her to have large blood and protein in her urine. Her electrolytes are Na 135, K 5.3, bil 16, urea 13.6, creatinine 132.

You suspect she has glomerulonephritis. What would you expect her C_3 and C_4 results to be?

    (i) C_3 normal C_4 normal
    (ii) C_3 low C_4 low
    (iii) C_3 low C_4 normal
    (iv) C_3 normal C_4 low
    (v) C_3 high C_4 high

14.18 You were asked to review a four-hour-old baby because of a swelling on the scalp. Which one of the following would suggest a cephalhaematoma as opposed to caput succedaneum?
        (i)   poorly defined outline
        (ii) caused by pressure
        (iii) still present at two weeks
        (iv) noticed at birth
        (v) swelling crosses the suture line

14.19 A three-hour-old baby who was born below the 3rd centile is being closely monitored for symptoms of hypoglycaemia.

Which of the following is not a symptom?

  (i)   cyanosis
  (ii) plethora
  (iii) respiratory distress
  (iv) temperature instability
  (v)   pallor

14.20 It is 10.00 p.m. and you are rung by the GP out of hours because he has a baby with a pyrexia. He says the temperature is 103.1°F.

What is this in centigrade?

  (i)   38.0°C
  (ii) 40.0°C
  (iii) 38.5°C
  (iv) 39.5°C
  (v)   39.0°C

14.21 A six-year-old boy is admitted with a short history of frequency. The SHO notices there is some swelling around the eyes and suspects nephrotic syndrome.

Which of the following is not consistent with the diagnosis?

  (i)   proteinuria
  (ii) hypoalbuminaemia
  (iii) hypertension
  (iv) generalized oedema
  (v)   hyperlipidaemia

14.22 A four-year-old boy comes in with a short illness and having not passed urine for 12 hours. On admission his urea is 9 and his creatinine is 150. Urine output continues to be very poor.

Which of the following is not a pre-renal cause?

  (i)   burns
  (ii) nephrotic syndrome
  (iii) acute gastroenteritis
  (iv) haemolytic–uraemic syndrome
  (v)   septicaemic shock

14.23 A six-month-old baby is being assessed for development. Tone seems all right and he is alert.

Which of the following reflexes would be normal at this age?

    (i)   Moro reflex
    (ii) asymmetric tonic neck reflex
    (iii) hand grasp
    (iv) parachute
    (v) plantar grasp

14.24 A seven-year-old is coming up for his three-monthly review. He was diagnosed as having cystic fibrosis four years ago. He also, on questioning, has some exercise intolerance which has been helped by the GP prescribing a beta agonist.

Which one of the following lung function tests best fits?

	FVC	FEV$_1$	PEF
Predicted	2.0	1.9	280
(i)	2.2	1.7	210
(ii)	1.6	1.1	200
(iii)	1.5	1.4	170
(iv)	1.7	1.8	250
(v)	1.9	1.0	160

14.25 You are referred a nine-year-old girl with short stature. Cardiovascular and respiratory systems are normal. Assessment of her pubertal development shows she has enlargement of the breast and areola areas but there is no separation in their contours. There is a sparse growth of slightly downy hair along the labia.

Her pubertal staging is:

	Breast	Pubic hair
(i)	II	III
(ii)	II	II
(iii)	III	III
(iv)	III	II
(v)	III	IV

14.26 You are asked to see a six-year-old boy who is causing disruption at school and home. During the consultation he doesn't sit still. When asked, his mother says he is sleeping no more than four hours a night.

What should be his typical sleep needs?

    (i)   12 hours
    (ii)   7 hours
    (iii) 11 hours
    (iv) 9 hours
    (v)   8 hours

14.27 You are reviewing the neonatal unit's yearly figures and one of the many calculations you have been asked to do is the neonatal mortality rate.

Which of the following is the correct calculation?

    (i)   deaths in 1st week of total births
    (ii)   deaths in 1st month of total births
    (iii) deaths in 1st week of live births
    (iv) deaths in 1st month of live births
    (v)   deaths in 1st month of total births (excluding lethal malformation)

14.28 You are reviewing a baby on the neonatal unit who is cyanotic with a heart murmur. An urgent echo shows that he has Fallot's tetralogy. The mother and father are both solicitors and you are explaining the cause of Fallot's. They understand the heart problem and wonder when it happened. You explain that it occurred during the embryonic stage of development.

This is up to what stage in pregnancy?

    (i)   7 weeks
    (ii)   8 weeks
    (iii) 9 weeks
    (iv) 10 weeks
    (v)   11 weeks

ANSWERS

14.1 **(a)** (v)

(b) Lateral hip X-ray.
Comment: Fit the diagnosis with the patient's age. He would need to be younger for Perthes' (four to eight years of age).

14.2 X-ray the rest of the leg.
Comment: Pathology may have been missed; for example, Ewing's sarcoma.

14.3 The first rise is transplacental IgG, which dips before the baby starts producing its own.

14.4 (iii)

0 – no movement
1 – slight movement
2 – movement, but not against gravity
3 – movement against gravity
4 – near normal
5 – normal

14.5 **(a)** (ii)

(b) Many places, commonly anterior to the ear or the middle of the neck.

14.6 **(a)** (i)

(b) The swelling will settle, leaving a palpable remnant only.

(c) No.
Comment: Congenital torsion is usually on the left and, unlike torsion in the older age group, the other testis does not need fixing.

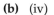

14.7 **(a)** (ii)

(b) (iv)

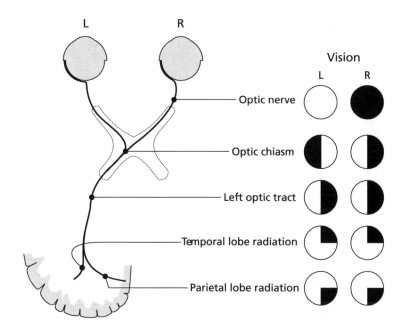

Comment: Whenever answering a question on visual pathways, draw the pathway.

14.8 No.

Comment: One WBC for 500 RBC = 214 000/500 = 428.

14.9 **(a)** (iii)

(b) Respiratory function using a spirometer.
Comment: Question **(b)** removes any uncertainty regarding question **(a)**.

14.10 Discitis; tumour.
Comment: In view of non-raised CRP it is difficult to put the answers in order.

14.11 (ii) $(14 \times 90)/(6 \times 7.5)$
Comment: Just make sure whether the O_2 is kPa or mmHg.

14.12 (iii)
Comment: 2.7 is the current recommendation.

14.13 (v) Some people will say up to a 100 but I believe 50 is generous enough.

14.14 **(a)** (v)

(b) (ii)   When do you believe you should mention this to parents?

14.15 **(a)** (ii)

(b) (iv)
Comment: Go through one generation at a time.

14.16 **(a)** (ii)

(b) (iv)
Comment: It could almost be any of them but ITP can follow a cold, so that is the right answer.

14.17 (ii)

14.18 (iii)
Comment: It may calcify and so last several weeks.

14.19 (ii)
Comment: This is cause, whereas the rest are effect.

14.20 (iv)
Comment: $C \to F$ = temperature $\times 9/5 + 32$.

14.21 (iii) Consistent with nephritic syndrome.
Comment: Renal cause.

14.22 (iv)

14.23 (ii)
Comment: It is worth preparing a table of development and reflexes as this is also very useful for Part II.

14.24 (ii) = mixed picture

14.25 (iv)

14.26 (iii)

14.27 (ii)
Comment: It is useful to know the different definitions.

14.28 (iii)

Exam 1

15

QUESTIONS

15.1 A cardiologist is reviewing a two-year-old with a systolic murmur. He is noted to have some soft dysmorphic features:

ECG – normal

Echo – mild supravalvular aortic stenosis

(a) What is the likely diagnosis?
   (i) Prader–Willi syndrome
   (ii) Angelman's syndrome
   (iii) cri du chat
   (iv) Williams' syndrome
   (v) Alagille's syndrome

(b) Give one other cardiac lesion.
   (i) coarctation
   (ii) peripheral pulmonary stenosis
   (iii) pulmonary atresia
   (iv) tetralogy of Fallot
   (v) transposition

(c) What blood test may be abnormal in the neonatal period?
   (i) hypercalcaemia
   (ii) hypocalcaemia
   (iii) hyperkalaemia
   (iv) hypokalaemia
   (v) hypoglycaemia

(d) What is the confirmatory test?
  - (i) chromosome analysis
  - (ii) FISH – chromosome 7
  - (iii) liver biopsy
  - (iv) FISH – chromosome 15
  - (v) FISH – chromosome 5

15.2 A 15-year-old is admitted with meningitis. While in hospital he has audiometry tests.

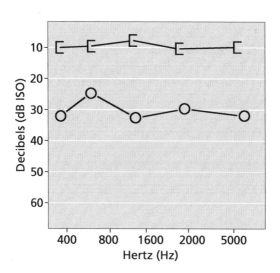

(a) Does he need an operation?

(b) Justify your answer.

15.3 A five-year-old with known renal tubular acidosis has the following test result: Bicarbonate loading – urine more alkaline

Which type of RTA does he have?

15.4 A boy presents to you in out-patients with a one-week history of a cough; he is also pyrexial. He has a history of frequent skin abscesses and intermittent diarrhoea.

(a) What would you expect his immunoglobulins to be (IgA, IgM, IgG)?

(b) What is the inheritance?
  (i) X-linked recessive
  (ii) X-linked dominant
  (iii) autosomal dominant
  (iv) autosomal recessive
  (v) mitochondrial

(c) Name one confirmatory test.

(d) What treatment may be required?

15.5 A newly diagnosed diabetic has high pre-breakfast blood sugars, but is also noted to be sweaty in the night.

(a) What is the diagnosis?

(b) What is the treatment plan?

15.6 A baby on the neonatal unit with prolonged jaundice is found to have a TSH of 150 mU/L.

Name two associated syndromes.

15.7 This is the family tree of a girl under your care. Her parents both have the same condition.

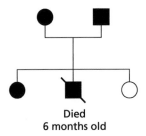

Died
6 months old

(a) What is the condition?

(b) What caused her brother's death?

15.8   A six-year-old presents to the department with a pyrexia and neck stiffness.

LP result:

RBC	21×10^6/L
WBC	264×10^6/L

Gram-positive diplococcus

(a)   What is the likely organism?
  (i)   meningococcus
  (ii)   listeria
  (iii) haemophilus
  (iv)   pneumococcus
  (v)   *E. coli*

(b)   Suggest an antibiotic.

(c)   What would you expect the glucose to be?

15.9   A two-year-old girl is admitted with a two-month history of polyuria and polydipsia. She also vomits intermittently and has gained weight:

On admission	glycosuria
Blood sugar	11.2 mmol/L
Blood gas	normal
Overnight	BMs 4–7 mmol/L
Next morning	blood sugar 4.6 mmol/L

(a)   What is the most likely diagnosis?
  (i)   diabetes mellitus
  (ii)   cranial diabetes insipidus
  (iii) nephrogenic diabetes insipidus
  (iv)   psychogenic polydipsia
  (v)   normal

(b)   What is the management?

15.10 A 6½-year-old is referred to you because of her short stature. The following results are available:

FBC	Normal
U&Es	Normal
GH	110 mU/L
TSH	Normal

(a) What is the likely diagnosis?

(b) What is the mode of inheritance?
- (i) autosomal recessive
- (ii) autosomal dominant
- (iii) X-linked dominant
- (iv) X-linked recessive
- (v) mitochondrial

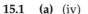
15.1 **(a)** (iv)

(b) (ii)

(c) (i)

(d) (iv)
Comment: I believe that all new information is collected on a card system. There are lots of conditions linked to cardiac conditions. If you record them all together then if you do not know the right answer you will know which are wrong.

15.2 **(a)** No (not with the information given).

(b) The tests show mild right conductive hearing loss. The worry in meningitis is sensorineuronal loss.

15.3 Proximal renal tubular acidosis.
Comment: Acid or base loading will not change the pH in distal renal tubular acidosis.

15.4 **(a)** All raised.

(b) (i)

(c) Nitroblue tetrazolium dye reduction test.

(d) Antibiotics, white cell transfusion, bone marrow transplant.
Comment: He has chronic granulomatous disease.

15.5 **(a)** Somogyi effect.

(b) Decrease evening insulin.
Comment: Too much insulin causes nocturnal hypoglycaemia with compensatory growth hormone and cortisol surges. As the influence of exogenous insulin diminishes, early-morning hyperglycaemia occurs.

15.6 Down's syndrome; Pendred's syndrome.

15.7 **(a)** Achondroplasia.

(b) Constrictive thoracic dystrophy.
Comment: Caused by the double dominant.

15.8 **(a)** (iv)

(b) Ceftriaxone, cefotaxime etc., or penicillin.

(c) Low/less than 40% of the blood glucose.
Comment: Remember the relationship between CSF and blood glucose.

15.9 **(a)** (iv)
(b) Gradual decrease in fluids.

Comment: Does not fit with diabetes as blood gas is normal and settles with no treatment. High glucose can be caused by glucose drinks.

15.10 **(a)** Laron dwarfism.

(b) (i)
Comment: End-organ growth hormone insensitivity.

Exam 2

QUESTIONS

16.1 This is the spirometer reading of an eight-year-old girl.

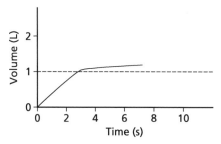

FVC   1.2 litres
FEF(25–75%)   40%

(a) What condition does she have?
   (i)   asthma
   (ii)   cystic fibrosis
   (iii)   pneumonia
   (iv)   fibrosing alveolitis
   (v)   pneumothorax

(b) What would you expect her FEV_1 to be?
   (i)   normal
   (ii)   slightly increased
   (iii)   slightly decreased
   (iv)   markedly decreased
   (v)   markedly increased

16.2 How old are these children?
- (i) 1 year
- (ii) 18 months
- (iii) 2 years
- (iv) 2½ years
- (v) 3 years
- (vi) 3½ years
- (vii) 4 years
- (viii) 4½ years
- (ix) 5 years
- (x) 5½ years
- (xi) 6 years

Give their age from the above list by their ability to do the following:

(a) Make a tower of five bricks.

(b) Copy a flight of stairs out of building blocks.

(c) Draw

○ ....

□ ....

△ _____

16.3 A four-year-old boy with a known hearing loss has the following test result:

Right	Rinne negative
Left	Rinne positive
Weber	right

(a) What hearing loss does he have?
- (i) bilateral conductive hearing loss
- (ii) right conductive hearing loss
- (iii) left conductive hearing loss
- (iv) right sensorineural loss
- (v) left sensorineural loss

(b) What is his bone conduction on the affected side?

16.4 Two unrelated families have had the same spontaneous mutation:

Family 1   Family 2

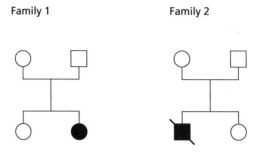

(a) What is the condition?

(b) What is the mode of inheritance?
    (i)   autosomal dominant
    (ii)   autosomal recessive
    (iii) X-linked recessive
    (iv) X-linked dominant
    (v)   mitochondrial

16.5 A 15-year-old girl with well-controlled diabetes starts drinking excessively and passing a lot of urine.

What is the underlying diagnosis?
    (i)   cranial diabetes insipidus
    (ii)   not taking her insulin
    (iii) DIDMOAD
    (iv) UTI
    (v)   nephrogenic diabetes insipidus

16.6 A 14-year-old child is causing concern because her standing height is tailing off the centiles. She is developmentally normal and well. She is also entering puberty.

(a) What is the likely underlying diagnosis?
    (i)   achondroplasia
    (ii)   Turner's syndrome
    (iii) hypochondroplasia
    (iv) rickets
    (v)   missed congenital adrenal hypoplasia

(b) How may this be confirmed clinically?

16.7 A school child is noticed to be jaundiced. The following results are obtained:

Bilirubin	120 μmol/L
Direct	110 μmol/L
Urinary coproporphyrins	normal with greater than 80% coproporphyrin 1

    (a) What is the likely diagnosis?
        (i)   hepatitis C
        (ii) Dubin–Johnson syndrome
        (iii) Gilbert's syndrome
        (iv) Crigler–Najjar syndrome
        (v)   Rotor's syndrome

    (b) What will the liver biopsy show?

16.8 A 3½-year-old is brought to you with obesity. He also has undescended testes. In the neonatal period he needed tube feeding.

    (a) What is the most likely diagnosis?

    (b) What are the two modes of inheritance?

    (c) Which mode is more common?

16.9 A 2½-year-old is referred to your clinic because of irritability and sweatiness. There has been poor weight gain in the last six months.

    (a) What is the diagnosis?
        (i)   cystic fibrosis
        (ii) TB
        (iii) hyperthyroidism
        (iv) Bartter's syndrome
        (v)   pseudo-Bartter's syndrome

    (b) Suggest a treatment.

    (c) What is the natural history?

16.10 An eight-year-old boy is under your care and is having a glycogen stimulation test.

Time (s)	GH (mU/L)	Cortisol (nmol/L)
0	6.4	93
30	5.4	270
60	2.6	187
90	1.1	120
120	2.8	125
180	7.2	184

(a) What does the test show?
  (i) normal
  (ii) GH normal, cortisol deficient
  (iii) GH deficient, cortisol normal
  (iv) both deficient
  (v) inadequate test

(b) What is your management plan?
  (i) repeat test
  (ii) give GH
  (iii) give cortisol
  (iv) give GH and cortisol
  (v) leave alone

16.1 **(a)** (i)

(b) (iv)
Comment: Look at Respiratory medicine chapter.

16.2 **(a)** (iii)

(b) (vii)

(c) (v, x, viii)
Comment: Unfortunately this just has to be learned!

16.3 **(a)** (ii)

(b) Normal.
Comment: Remember Rinne negative is always the abnormal ear.

16.4 **(a)** Incontinentia pigmenti.

(b) (iv)
Comment: There are a few males with this condition but most do not survive.

16.5 (iii)
Comment: Diabetes insipidus is the diagnosis but the above is the underlying diagnosis.

DI = diabetic insipidus
DM = diabetes mellitus
OA = optic atrophy
D   = deafness

16.6 **(a)** (ii)

(b) Sitting height.
Comment: Shortening of limbs becomes more obvious at puberty. Sitting height is nearer normal.

16.7 **(a)** (ii)

(b) Normal.
Comment: If you do not know the answer then rule out the ones with unconjugated jaundice, then you are only guessing from two.

16.8 **(a)** Prader–Willi syndrome.

(b) Paternal deletion; maternal disomy.

(c) Paternal deletion.
Comment: Paternal deletion/maternal disomy = Prader–Willi syndrome. Paternal disomy/maternal deletion = Angelman's syndrome.

16.9 **(a)** (iii)

(b) Carbimazole propranolol.

(c) The child will grow out of it.

16.10 **(a)** (iv)

(b) (iv) GH supplementation: one i.m. injection six days a week. Cortisol supplementation: ⅔ morning, ⅓ evening; increased with illness and early admission if vomiting.
Comment: **(b)** tells you the answer to **(a)**

Exam 3

17

17.1 An eight-year-old boy is admitted with a painful left ankle associated with a limp. There was also some pain in the left wrist. On examination he looks well and is apyrexial. There is no obvious swelling. The pain settled with ibuprofen. There was a history of a mild sore throat about three weeks ago:

Hb	12.4 g/dL
WCC	10.6×10^9/L
Platelets	474×10^9/L
ESR	56×10^9/L
Rh factor	<20 mm/h
Anti-nuclear antibodies	negative

He is still well one year later.

Give the most likely diagnosis.
- (i) monoarticular arthritis
- (ii) reactive arthropathy
- (iii) sprained ankle
- (iv) Still's disease
- (v) streptococcal septic arthritis

17.2 You are asked to review a five-year-old girl with a nine-month history of tenderness over the breasts. She is also noted to have developed some pubic hair in the last two months. She is on the 97th centile but her bone age is not advanced. The following results are available:

TSH	2.2 mU/L	
Oestradiol	400 pmol/L	
Prolactin	131 (normal 0–450) mU/L	
LHRH test time (min)	**LH (U/L)**	**FSH (U/L)**
0	<1	40
30	22.0	19.2
60	14.3	19.9

(a) What do the tests show?

(b) What other investigation is necessary and why?

17.3 A four-year-old child with a positive family history of spherocytosis undergoes an osmotic fragility test:

Mean cell fragility fresh 4.6 g/L NaCl (4–4.45)

post-incubation 6.6 g/L NaCl (4.65–5.9)

Has the child got spherocytosis?

17.4 A two-year-old boy is admitted with a swollen face and abdominal distension of seven days' standing. He has been treated for a sore throat:

Hb	12.2 g/dl
WCC	13.9×10^9/L
Platelets	547×10^9/L
Urea	3.3 mmol/L
Sodium	138 mmol/L
BP	120/70 mmHg
Albumin	16 g/L
Urine protein	+++

(a) What is the likely diagnosis?
- (i) haemolytic uraemic syndrome
- (ii) Epstein–Barr
- (iii) nephritic syndrome
- (iv) nephrotic syndrome
- (v) UTI

(b) What is the initial treatment?

(c) What is the long-term course?

17.5 On holiday, a five-year-old presents with haematuria. There is no history of illness and he is well.

Urine:

RBC	Uncountable
WBC	<2006/L
No organisms seen	

Blood:

Hb	12.4 g/dL
WCC	10.1×10^9/L
Platelets	232×10^9/L
Sodium	136 mmol/L
Potassium	4.6 mmol/L
Urea	3.2 mmol/L
Albumin	44 g/L

(a) Give three possible diagnoses.

(b) Name three further observations/investigations.

17.6   You are reviewing a nine-year-old in clinic whom you have been treating with vasopressin for four years. You have just plotted his height and weight (see chart):

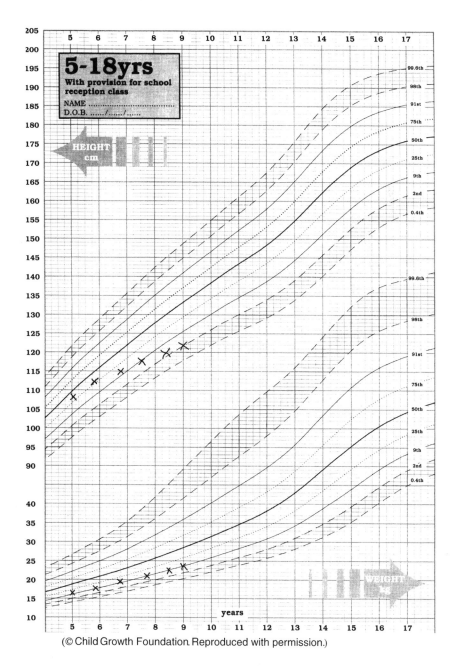

(© Child Growth Foundation. Reproduced with permission.)

(a) Give a likely diagnosis for the growth chart.
   (i)   inadequate vasopressin
   (ii) diabetes mellitus
   (iii) hypothyroidism
   (iv) coeliac disease
   (v)   growth hormone deficiency

(b) Give an underlying diagnosis.

(c) Name two other tests you should do.

17.7 A 10-year-old boy is admitted to A&E unable to walk and complaining of pain in his thighs. He has previously been fit and well:

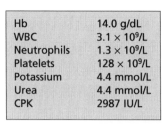

Hb	14.0 g/dL
WBC	3.1×10^9/L
Neutrophils	1.3×10^9/L
Platelets	128×10^9/L
Potassium	4.4 mmol/L
Urea	4.4 mmol/L
CPK	2987 IU/L

(a) What is the likely diagnosis?
  (i)   Duchenne's disease
  (ii)   Ewing's sarcoma
  (iii) viral myositis
  (iv)   dermatomyositis
  (v)   steroid-induced myositis

(b) What is the prognosis?

17.8 The following results are from a sample of milk:

Protein	3.3 g/dL
Fat	3.7 g/dL
Sodium	24 mmol/L

What kind of milk is it?
  (i)   breast milk
  (ii)   formula milk
  (iii) goat's milk
  (iv)   cow's milk
  (v)   pre-term formula

17.9 A three-year-old boy, who has had recurrent otitis media, is now having difficulties hearing the television. If his right and left ears are equally affected, what would you expect his Rinne and Weber tests to show?

	Rinne left	Rinne right	Weber
(i)	positive	negative	right
(ii)	positive	positive	central
(iii)	negative	positive	central
(iv)	negative	negative	central
(v)	negative	negative	right

17.10 A 12-year-old, known to have a VSD, has a cardiac catheterization:

RA	81
RV	80
Pulmonary	82
LA	96
LV	90
Aorta	90

What does it show?

17.1 (ii)
Comment: Good response to ibuprofen with no return of symptoms. The ESR can be raised.

17.2 (a) Pubertal response to LHRH stimulation test.

(b) MRI, as central cause indicated.
Comment: Remember, if LH/FSH is pre-pubertal, you would have to scan adrenals and ovaries.

17.3 Yes.
Comment: You do not even need to know the test to answer this, as the result is outside the normal range.

17.4 (a) (iv)

(b) High-dose prednisolone.

(c) Relapsing, but usually remains steroid sensitive.

17.5 (a) Renal stone; nephritic syndrome; viral cystitis.

(b) Kidney/ureter/bladder X-ray; urine protein; blood pressure.
Comment: There is no test for viral cystitis so concentrate on the other two diagnoses.

17.6 (a) (v)

(b) Histiocytosis X.

(c) ACTH, TSH studies.
Comment: This is a good example of how (b) and (c) give clues to (a).

17.7 (a) (iii)

(b) He will get better.
Comment: CPK is high enough for muscular dystrophy but unlikely because of the acute onset.

17.8 (iv)
Comment: This is one of those questions where it is very difficult to rule out any of the answers so you may just end up guessing.

17.9 (iv)
Comment: Look at the Audiometry chapter.

17.10 Eisenmenger's syndrome through the VSD.
Comment: You would lose marks for just Eisenmenger's syndrome.

Themed
questions

18

HOW TO ANSWER THEMED QUESTIONS

It is quite easy to get confused with so many answers.

I believe doing them in your head is a sure way of making a mistake.

It is worth doing each part as a separate question as they are not related, so why not use a different colour for each when looking for wrong answers?

It is also possible to think of the diagnosis without looking at the answers when you know the theme.

Finally, remember that the parts can have the same answer.

18.1 Theme – Syndromes

(i)	Williams'	(ix)	McCune–Albright
(ii)	Down's	(x)	tubular sclerosis
(iii)	Turner's	(xi)	Alagille's
(iv)	Noonan's	(xii)	Angelman's
(v)	Marfan's	(xiii)	cri du chat
(vi)	homocystinuria	(xiv)	Alport's
(vii)	neurofibromatosis	(xv)	Edward's
(viii)	congenital adrenal hyperplasia	(xvi)	Patau's

(a) You are reviewing a six-year-old girl with mild learning problems and short stature. The baby had a murmur noted in the neonatal period. The cardiologist diagnosed a pulmonary valve stenosis but it has settled with no treatment.

(b) You are following up a toddler who in the neonatal period was picked up as having peripheral artery stenosis and also some abnormal biochemistry results.

(c) A four-year-old girl is referred to you because of precocious puberty. The GP has checked the electrolytes and they are normal. The examination is unremarkable apart from a large birthmark and a few smaller ones.

(d) You are asked to review a newborn baby girl. Antenatally she was noted to have a horseshoe kidney. On examination she is very growth retarded; she also has rockerbottom feet.

18.2   Theme – Cardiac catheterization

	RA	RV	PA	LA	LV	A
(i)	65	65	65	95	95	95
(ii)	65	65	95	95	95	65
(iii)	65	75	75	95	95	95
(iv)	65	65	65	95	95	85
(v)	65	65	65	95	85	85
(vi)	75	75	75	94	94	94

Which of the above is consistent with:

(a)   A cyanotic newborn with no murmur?

(b)   A baby with a localized murmur at the LSE?

(c)   An ejection systolic murmur radiating to the back?

18.3 Theme – Chromosomes

(i)	1	(xiii)	13
(ii)	2	(xiv)	14
(iii)	3	(xv)	15
(iv)	4	(xvi)	16
(v)	5	(xvii)	17
(vi)	6	(xviii)	18
(vii)	7	(xix)	19
(viii)	8	(xx)	20
(ix)	9	(xxi)	21
(x)	10	(xxii)	22
(xi)	11	(xxiii)	X
(xii)	12	(xxiv)	Y

(a) You are reviewing a four-year-old with increasing weight which the mother is surprised about as she needed nasogastric feeds as a neonate.

(b) You are reviewing a seven-year-old who has just started having seizures. He also has some learning difficulties.

(c) You are seeing a seven-year-old girl with moderate bleeding problems. Her results are as follows:

Bleeding time – increased

PT – normal

APPT – slightly increased

TT – normal

(d) You are reviewing a two-week-old baby with hepatitis. Two relatives are under the respiratory physician for emphysema.

(i)	A	(vii)	K
(ii)	B_6	(viii)	copper
(iii)	B_{12}	(ix)	folate
(iv)	C	(x)	iron
(v)	D	(xi)	zinc
(vi)	E	(xii)	calcium

Which of the above are the following children most at risk of being deficient?

(a) A six-month-old baby who is fully breast-fed and the mother is asking for advice about weaning (give two).

(b) An eight-month-old who is thriving but seems not to be very hungry. On questioning he is drinking five to six bottles of doorstep milk a day (give one).

(c) A 15-year-old who is on an elemental diet for his Crohn's disease. He has had two operations for strictures (give two).

(d) A 10-year-old girl who, along with her mother, has been a strict vegan for the last two years (give one).

18.5   Theme – Eye changes

      (i)   chorioretinitis
     (ii)   cataracts
   (iii)   corneal clouding
   (iv)   upward dislocation of lens
    (v)   downward dislocation of lens
   (vi)   retinitis pigmentosa
  (vii)   retinopathy of prematurity
 (viii)   glaucoma
   (ix)   papilloedema

Which eye change is most likely?

(a)   An ex-premature 26/40 baby is being reviewed when you notice nystagmus. He is also noted to have a small head and a subsequent CT shows calcification. What is the most likely cause of the nystagmus?

(b)   You are asked to see an eight-year-old boy with some learning difficulties as a possible Marfan's syndrome. However, you feel that the child probably has homocystinuria. What eye signs would confirm this?

(i)	FBC	(ix)	CRP
(ii)	FBC + film	(x)	amylase
(iii)	U&Es	(xi)	glucose
(iv)	U&Es + chloride	(xii)	sweat test
(v)	arterial gas	(xiii)	anti-endomysial antibodies
(vi)	LFTs	(xiv)	IgE and RAST
(vii)	TFTs	(xv)	Group and Coombs
(viii)	$C_3 C_4$	(xvi)	bilirubin Q–bone marrow

Which single test will be most helpful in confirming a diagnosis?

(a) A 10-year-old girl presents with abdominal pain and diarrhoea. She is noted to have a node in her neck and her BP is 110/70. Her urine has 3+ blood and 3+ protein.

(b) A newborn baby is the product of the third pregnancy of a 28-year-old Caucasian. The mother is O rhesus positive and there is jaundice noted at 15 hours.

(c) A six-year-old child presents with abdominal pain and diarrhoea. You notice that she has a palpable spleen. Her mother says she and her sister had splenectomies as teenagers.

(d) A three-week-old presents with increasingly forceful vomits. There is no weight loss and he is still hungry.

(e) You are seeing a 15-year-old boy with severe abdominal pain. In the past he has had a normal appendix removed. During this episode he notices his stools are fatty. He is tender and pale but otherwise well.

(f) You have been seeing a three-year-old in clinic for six months. He has a history of diarrhoea and asthma. You notice his weight is beginning to tail off.

(g) A 25-weeker is now eight weeks old and is on 0.2 L/min of oxygen. He has twice failed to wean from this level and there is talk of home oxygen.

18.7   Theme – Arterial gases

	pH	PCO₂	PO₂	HCO₃	BE
(i)	7.41	56	70	32	+9
(ii)	7.45	30	60	33	+11
(iii)	7.48	22	130	25	−10
(iv)	7.29	46	29	19.2	−4.4
(v)	7.37	33.8	46.5	20.5	−4.8
(vi)	7.25	40	60	15	−9.0
(vii)	7.10	25	80	5	−16.0

Which gases fit the clinical case?

(a)   You are called by A&E, who have a 15-year-old who is said to have ingested a mixture of aspirin and paracetamol two hours earlier. She is previously known to have been in with alcohol intoxication.

(b)   A 25-weeker on SCBU has been stable for the past two hours when suddenly the sats drop to the 70s and the blood pressure drops to 27/15, mean 19. Increasing the oxygen from 60% to 100% doesn't seem to help. There is a bilateral good air entry and cold light is normal.

(c)   An ex-prem of 25 weeks is still in oxygen at 38 weeks. The X-ray is consistent with chronic lung disease. As he is stable, he is due to go home.

(i)	6 weeks	(viii)	2 years
(ii)	3 months	(ix)	2½ years
(iii)	6 months	(x)	3 years
(iv)	9 months	(xi)	3½ years
(v)	12 months	(xii)	4 years
(vi)	15 months	(xiii)	4½ years
(vii)	18 months	(xiv)	5 years

How old are these children?

(a) Tom can kick a ball and has just started riding a tricycle. He can put two words together but will not say his name.

(b) Jane is turning to your voice and will sit alone for a few minutes. She is also becoming shy to strangers. She will eat with her fingers but not drink from a cup. She has not started saying 'mama', 'dada' yet.

(c) Peter copies a circle and is just beginning to hop. He cannot draw a cross yet.

(d) Jack has lost his stepping reflex but still has his Moro and tonic neck reflexes.

(e) Becky has lost her stepping, Moro and grasp reflexes but has a Galant's reflex. She doesn't have a parachute reaction.

(f) Amy can build stairs and copy a square.

18.9 Theme – Milks

/100 ml	Energy (kcal)	Protein (g)	Ca (mg)	Na (mg)
(i)	70	1.8	22	29
(ii)	80	2.4	100	41
(iii)	70	1.3	35	15
(iv)	67	3.4	124	52
(v)	68	1.5	56	26
(vi)	75	1.0	70	80

Which is consistent with the following milks?

(a) Cow's milk.

(b) Breast milk and fortifier.

(c) Premature formula.

18.10 Theme – Cardiac catheterizations

	RA	RV	PA	LA	LV	A
(i)	58	60	59	95	94	95
(ii)	58	70	70	95	95	95
(iii)	75	75	75	95	95	95
(iv)	60	60	60	95	85	85
(v)	60	60	75	95	95	95
(vi)	60	60	60	95	94	87

Which of the above is most consistent with the following diagnosis?

(a) ASD.

(b) Aortic stenosis.

(c) Primary pulmonary hypertension with patent duct.

(d) Pulmonary stenosis.

(e) Tetralogy of Fallot with cyanosis.

(i)	Kawasaki's syndrome	(ix)	rheumatic fever
(ii)	infectious mononucleosis	(x)	herpes
		(xi)	TB
(iii)	erythema infectiosum	(xii)	inflammatory bowel disease
(iv)	measles	(xiii)	HSP
(v)	German measles	(xiv)	meningococcal septicaemia
(vi)	pityriasis rosea	(xv)	roseola infantum
(vii)	scabies		
(viii)	urticaria		

Which diagnosis is most likely?

(a) You are reviewing a three-year-old on the ward who was admitted 24 hours ago with pyrexia. The urine is clear and examination on admission was unremarkable. On review she now has a widespread macular rash and her temperature seems to be settling.

(b) A four-year-old child is admitted with an urticarial rash on the lower limbs and some pain in the right knee. Over the next 12 hours the child complains of some abdominal pain and some of the rash becomes non-blanching.

(c) A six-year-old child is admitted with pyrexia and is slightly irritable. On examination she is snuffly with what looks like numerous flea bites.

(d) A little girl is admitted with a sore mouth and a macular rash. Over the course of time several lesions appear like targets and you suspect it is erythema multiforme.

(i)   maple syrup urine disease
(ii)   acute hereditary tyrosinaemia
(iii)   non-ketotic hyperglycaemia
(iv)   urea cycle disorder
(v)   propionic acidaemia
(vi)   galactosaemia
(vii)   glycogen storage disease Type 1
(viii) pyruvate dehydrogenase deficiency
(ix)   MCAD
(x)   mitochondrial disease
(xi)   Menke's disease
(xii)   Smith–Lemli–Opitz syndrome

Which diagnosis is most likely?

(a)   A four-month-old baby is seen in out-patients because of worries about development. The neonatal period shows a history of poor temperature. On examination there is abnormal tone and hair.

(b)   You are reviewing a baby on SCBU with continuing severe hypoglycaemia. Some of the results show a marked lactic acidosis, hyperuricaemia and hyperlipidaemia. Abdominal ultrasound shows a large liver although it is difficult to palpate.

(c)   A seven-day-old is rushed into A&E with vomiting and he has lost more than 10% of weight. He looks septic and this is proven to have *E. coli* with associated UTI. The liver is palpable.

18.1 **(a)** (iv)
Comment: Originally called male Turner's syndrome. Also affects girls.

(b) (xi or i)
Comment: Sorry, there will only be one answer in the exam.

(c) (ix)

(d) (xv)
Comment: Horseshoe kidney also occurs in Turner's syndrome.

18.2 **(a)** (ii)

(b) (iii)

(c) (i)
Comment: Remember – draw a box and work out what you are looking for with each diagnosis.

18.3 **(a)** (xv)

(b) (xii)

(c) (xiv)

(d) (xvi)
Comment: Worth a card as over time you will now collect numerous syndromes with their associated chromosome. Very easy to write questions.

18.4 **(a)** (v and vii)

(b) (x)

(c) (iii and v)

(d) (iii)
Comment: Terminal ileum.

18.5 **(a)** (i)

(b) (v)
Comment: Homocystinuria – low intelligence so lens down.

18.6 **(a)** (viii)

(b) (xv)

(c) (ii)

(d) (iv)

(e) (x)

(f) (xii)

(g) (i)
Comment: With each of these try and think of the diagnosis and then the test.

18.7 **(a)** (iii)

(b) (iv)

(c) (i)
Comment: For all of these try and decide what each column should do before looking.

18.8 **(a)** (viii)

(b) (iii)

(c) (x)

(d) (ii)

(e) (iii)

(f) (xiii)
Comment: Draw a chart of development – this will be very useful for the clinical.

18.9 **(a)** (iv)

(b) (ii)

(c) (ii)
Comment: (i) pre-term breast; (ii) breast and fortifier or Nutriprem; (iii) term milk; (iv) cow; (v) SMA; (vi) made up.

18.10 **(a)** (iii)

(b) (i)

(c) (vi)

(d) (i)

(e) (iv)
Comment: Hope you have drawn the boxes.

18.11 **(a)** (xv)

(b) (xiii)

(c) (xiv)

(d) (x)
Comment: Did you need the answers?

18.12 **(a)** (xi)

(b) (vii)

(c) (vi)

Practice exam

19

19.1 You are called to SCBU, where a septic 28-weeker 1.5 kg is on a ventilator. He is running a base deficit of −9 despite fluid boluses. It is now affecting ventilation needs so it is decided to treat him with 4.2% HCO_3.

How much is needed for a 1/2 correction?
  - (i) 4 ml
  - (ii) 9 ml
  - (iii) 2 ml
  - (iv) 2.25 ml
  - (v) 4.5 ml

19.2 You are reviewing a six-year-old boy with a one-week history of non-productive cough. He has an intermittent temperature and crackles at the left base. The X-ray shows some shadowing. You take an FBC and culture: Hb 9.3, WCC 13.6, 30% neutrophils.

Which antibiotic is likely to be most use?
  - (i) oral augmentin
  - (ii) i.v. augmentin
  - (iii) oral erythromycin
  - (iv) i.v. erythromycin
  - (v) i.v. cephalosporin

19.3 You are seeing a nine-year-old girl with a two-day history of initially diarrhoea then bile-stained vomit. She has had no vomiting for 24 hours but some abdominal pain. There are 35 WCC in the urine. The bowel sounds are present but you suspect she has appendicitis.

Which of the following WCC would fit with the diagnosis?
- (i)   3
- (ii)   7
- (iii)   10
- (iv)   20
- (v)   any of the above

19.4 You are reviewing the routine bloods of a 12-week-old 24-weeker. She was on TPN for three weeks and is now on EBM.

The following results are available:

Hb	9.6
Platelets	265
Ca	2.2
Reticulocytes	4.2
Alkaline phosphatase	950
Phosphate	1.1
GT	250

What further investigation would be most helpful?

- (i)   wrist X-ray
- (ii)   split bilirubin
- (iii)   LFTs
- (iv)   bilirubin
- (v)   urinary phosphate

19.5 You are reviewing four siblings because a cousin has died suddenly. The post mortem is normal and prolonged QT is suspected. You have the following results:

	Age	QT
Child A	2 weeks	0.46 s
Child B	3 years	0.41 s
Child C	6 years	0.46 s
Child D	10 years	0.38 s

How many have prolonged QT?

  (i)   0
  (ii)   1
  (iii)   2
  (iv)   3
  (v)   4

19.6 You are writing guidelines for resuscitation. How many ml/kg is right for the treatment of hypoglycaemia for infants?

  (i)   1 ml/kg of 10%
  (ii)   5 ml/kg of 10%
  (iii)   5 ml/kg of 50%
  (iv)   1 ml/kg of 50%
  (v)   1 ml/kg of 25%

19.7 A 10-year-old boy is admitted with bruises and petechiae. An FBC reveals ITP.

Which of the following would suggest a need for treatment?

  (i)   a three-week history
  (ii)   a two-day history
  (iii)   a platelet count of 1
  (iv)   bleeding from the mouth
  (v)   a bone marrow confirming the diagnosis

19.8 You are doing a first-day check and don't think there is a red reflex. Your registrar agrees with you. Which of the following is not likely?

    (i)   glaucoma
    (ii)   cataract
    (iii) retinoblastoma
    (iv) chorioretinitis
    (v)   none of above

19.9 Blood tests.

    (i)   FBC
    (ii)   CRP
    (iii)   U&Es
    (iv)   LFTs
    (v)   TFTs
    (vi)   PCR
    (vii) Bone profile
   (viii) chloride
    (ix)   blood sugar
    (x)   blood culture
    (xi)   clotting
    (xii) paracetamol levels
   (xiii) gas

Pick your first-choice test.

(a) A 12-year-old boy comes in on a Friday night having taken up to 20 paracetamol tablets the night before.

(b) A six-week-old baby is losing weight and seems to be hyper-alert and jittery.

(c) A 12-week-old ex-25-weeker has a normal gamma GT but a markedly raised alkaline phosphatase.

19.10 A three-year-old child has had confirmed shigella, has come in with deterioration and is shut down. His urea and creatinine are raised.

What is the likely diagnosis?
- (i) haemolytic uraemic syndrome
- (ii) shigella septicaemia
- (iii) dehydration
- (iv) pre-renal failure
- (v) none of the above

19.11 You are asked to see a baby with microcephaly on the labour ward.

Which of the following is unlikely?
- (i) maternal PKU
- (ii) PKU
- (iii) CMV
- (iv) rubella
- (v) none of the above

19.12 You are seeing this baby on the postnatal wards and clinically you think Turner's, heart sounds and femorals are normal. Which one of the following is not associated with this condition?

- (i) coarctation
- (ii) central infertility
- (iii) horseshoe kidney
- (iv) normal life expectancy
- (v) leukaemia

19.1 (v) $1/3 \times 1.5 \times 9 = 4.5$ ml (always look to see the concentration).

19.2 (iii) This picture fits with atypical pneumonia.

19.3 (v) The white count is not specific in appendicitis but it should be over 70% neutrophils.

19.4 (ii) Her GT suggests there is cholestasis.

19.5 (ii) QT is normal up to 0.44 but in neonates it can be up to 0.48.

19.6 (ii) No longer use 25% or 50%.

19.7 (iv)
Comment: Often the lowest count is on admission and guidance for treatment is bleeding.

19.8 (iv) This would have a red reflex.

19.9 **(a)** (xi)

(b) (v)

(c) (vii)
Comment: Come up with a diagnosis first.

19.10 (i)

19.11 (ii) This will cause microcephaly over time.

19.12 (ii) Streaked ovaries.

Practice exam long questions

20

The secret is to use the description to create the three-dimensional picture. Read the question, underlining anything that you feel is relevant. At the same time write diagnoses down the side that come to mind and then cross out any that stop being relevant.

20.1 Peter was born at 41 weeks' gestation and weighed 4.3 kg. His head circumference was 37 cm. He is the fourth baby of a Caucasian couple. They have two boys and a girl.

There was a fetal tachycardia with some decelerations. His Apgar scores were 9 and 9 and following a normal first examination he was discharged.

At six months of age he was admitted during the morning because his mother was unable to wake him. He had vomited the previous night.

On examination his temperature is 39°C. His pupils are small but reactive. There are no herpetic lesions or rash. His chest is clear and abdomen soft. His coma assessment is as follows:

No verbal response

Eyes react to pain

He flexes to pain

(a) What is his initial modified Glasgow Coma Scale?
  (i) 4
  (ii) 5
  (iii) 6
  (iv) 7
  (v) 8

(b) What is the most important initial test?
  (i) blood glucose
  (ii) arterial gas
  (iii) FBC
  (iv) U&Es
  (v) blood culture

An i.v.i. is set up and bloods are taken and the following results are available:

Na	147
K	5.6
U	15.7
HCO_3	15
Glu	0.5
FBC	clotted

Treatment is started.

PASS ✓

(c) Which of the following is the most important initial treatment?
- (i) saline bolus
- (ii) dextrose bolus
- (iii) broad-spectrum antibiotic
- (iv) rectal paracetamol
- (v) aciclovir

At 12.30 he starts fitting and is initially treated with diazepam. However, the fits continue and a decision is made to ventilate and transfer.

His first arterial gas shows:

pH	7.266
pCO_2	30.4
pO_2	176
HCO_3	17.8
BE	−8.4
Blood glucose	13.2

(d) What type of gas is this?
- (i) metabolic acidosis
- (ii) respiratory acidosis
- (iii) partially compensated metabolic acidosis
- (iv) mixed acidosis
- (v) partially compensated respiratory alkalosis

Prior to transfer, he has a normal CT scan and you have started him on both aciclovir and ceftriaxone.

(e) Which of the following is most likely?
- (i) sepsis
- (ii) non-accidental injury
- (iii) herpes encephalopathy
- (iv) metabolic disorder
- (v) drug ingestion

20.2 John was a normal term delivery with good Apgar scores. He was doing well until six months, when he was admitted unrousable and hypoglycaemic. This was very resistant to treatment and he required ventilation for 20 days. His diagnosis on discharge from the regional intensive care unit was glutaric aciduria Type II.

(a) Which of the following tests is used to confirm this diagnosis?
  (i) paired blood and urine amino acids
  (ii) liver biopsy
  (iii) white cell studies
  (iv) fibroblast culture
  (v) muscle biopsy

Over the next few weeks his tone increases, so it is decided that baclofen should be started. He continues to have severe seizures which need control with both lamotrigine and clonazepam.

At the age of nine months his seizures are well controlled and he is gastrostomy fed.

He has frequent admissions over the next two years with seizures. When he is about three, he comes in fitting.

(b) What weight is he?
  (i) 11 kg
  (ii) 12 kg
  (iii) 13 kg
  (iv) 14 kg
  (v) 15 kg

The ambulance staff have given him rectal diazepam and, as he has been fitting for 30 minutes, you decide to give him i.v. lorazepam.

(c) What is the correct dose for this?
  (i) 0.1 mg/kg
  (ii) 0.25 mg/kg
  (iii) 500 µg/kg
  (iv) 1 mg/kg
  (v) 5 mg/kg

(d) After the lorazepam how long do you wait before considering paraldehyde?
- (i)   1 minute
- (ii)   2 minutes
- (iii)   5 minutes
- (iv)   8 minutes
- (v)   10 minutes

Unfortunately he continues to fit so you decide to give him thiopentone and intubate him.

(e) The correct tube size is:
- (i)   3½
- (ii)   4
- (iii)   4½
- (iv)   5
- (v)   5½

20.3 Jessica was born by emergency section after a fetal tachycardia. She had a history of ruptured membranes for 30 hours. She responded to bag and mask and was transported to SCBU in 40% oxygen. She was noted to have a single umbilical artery. A UAC was inserted and a bolus of saline was given. Her first capillary gas was:

pH	6.96
pCO_2	16 kPa
pO_2	5.5 kPa
HCO_3	16.3
BE	−9.8

(a) Which of the following best describes the gas?
   (i) metabolic acidosis
   (ii) metabolic acidosis with hypoxia
   (iii) mixed acidosis with hypoxia
   (iv) mixed acidosis
   (v) metabolic alkalosis

The baby is intubated and surfactant is given. UVC is inserted and the X-ray suggests surfactant deficiency. After two boli of saline dopamine and dobutamine were started. Four hours later the gas is:

pH	7.322
pCO_2	3.6 kPa
pO_2	8 kPa
HCO_3	16
BE	−11.3

(b) What does this gas show?
   (i) compensated respiratory alkalosis
   (ii) compensated respiratory acidosis
   (iii) compensated metabolic alkalosis
   (iv) compensated metabolic acidosis
   (v) mixed acidosis

Four hours later the pH has deteriorated to 7.18 and so the ventilator is increased and a ½ correction of bicarbonate is given. She starts having fits shortly afterwards and is loaded with phenobarbital and then clonazepam.

At 24 hours she is in 100% oxygen with a mean airway pressure of 14. Her arterial oxygen is 9.3.

(c) What is her oxygen index?
   (i)   10
   (ii) 15
   (iii) 20
   (iv) 25
   (v)   30

20.4 John is born at 39 weeks by emergency section for meconium and failure to progress. He came out crying with good Apgar scores. Initially he went to the wards but very quickly started grunting and within 2 hours was ventilated.

The X-ray was consistent with meconium aspiration; however, the CRP was raised up to 320 and the blood culture grew *Listeria*.

(a) What do the bacteria look like?
  (i)   Gram-positive cocci
  (ii) Gram-negative cocci
  (iii) Gram-positive rod
  (iv) Gram-negative rod
  (v)   spirochaetes

(b) How long does he need antibiotics for?
  (i)   5 days
  (ii) 7 days
  (iii) 10 days
  (iv) 14 days
  (v)   21 days

20.5 Jane was born at 33 weeks in good condition with Apgar scores of 10 and 10. She has a history of prolonged rupture of membrane and at 1.2 kg is on the 0.4th centile. Because of the prolonged rupture she is screened. The following results are obtained:

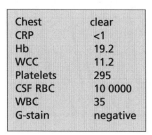

Chest	clear
CRP	<1
Hb	19.2
WCC	11.2
Platelets	295
CSF RBC	10 0000
WBC	35
G-stain	negative

After 48 hours the cultures come back negative.

(a) Do you:
   (i)   stop antibiotics
   (ii) continue for 5 days
   (iii) continue for 7 days
   (iv) continue for 10 days
   (v)   continue for 14 days

Over the next few days she gets on to full feeds and is doing well. However, on day eight she spikes a temperature and starts grunting. She is screened and put on second-line antibiotics.

The following results are available:

Day	8	9	10
CRP	11	14	34
Hb	17		
WCC	13		
Platelets	300		
Blood culture	Gram-positive cocci after 36 hours		

(b) What is the significance of the culture?

    (i)   contamination

    (ii)   *Staphylococcus aureus*

    (iii) Group B streptococcus

    (iv) coagulase-negative staphylococcus

    (v)   *E. coli*

She continues to deteriorate and is therefore transferred to the teaching centre and undergoes a laparotomy. They remove the right colon and appendix although it has perforated it looks healthy. There is nil else to find. After the operation she improves and her stomas are working.

By day 29 she is fully orally fed and growing. She is off antibiotics. You get the following report from the cytogenetics: No CF mutations detected. The mutations tested cover 90% of local mutations.

(c) What is the risk of missing CF?

    (i)   0%

    (ii)   0.01%

    (iii) 0.1%

    (iv) 1%

    (v)   10%

20.1 **(a)** (iii)

(b) (i)
Comment: Although probably septic because of his age, you need his glucose result.

(c) (ii)
Comment: Shows the importance of underlying the abnormal results.

(d) (iii)

(e) (i)
Comment: (iii) and (iv) are both possible but with the pyrexia the hypoglycaemia is most likely secondary to sepsis.

20.2 **(a)** (iv)

(b) (iv)

(c) (i)

(d) (iii)

(e) (iii)
Comment: These are all APLS questions – you need to have been on it to be a registrar so why wait?

20.3 **(a)** (iv) Cannot comment on the O_2 as capillary gas.

(b) (iv)

(c) (iii) $(100 \times 14)/(9.3 \times 7.5)$

20.4 **(a)** (iv)

(b) (iv)

20.5 **(a)** (i)

(b) (iv) Contamination if grown at birth.

(c) (iv) Two chromosomes – covered 90% of mutations each so missed 10%:

$10\% \times 10\% = 1\%$.

Index

63(66) indicates the locator for a question followed in brackets by the locator for its answer. The reader will often find the entry only located in the answer. 75(HH) refers to a 'helpful hint'.

PASS ✔

Index